PILLARS
OF DENTAL
SUCCESS

By:

Mark A. Costes, DDS

This book is dedicated to my parents,
Percy and Asuncion Costes. Everything that I
have and everything that I am I owe to you.
I love you both very much.

CONTENTS

FOREWORD

BY STEVE BEULIGMAN, DDS

Dentistry in the United States, in fact, our health-care system as a whole, is under siege from many forces. What is under attack is nothing less than the doctor–patient relationship—the founding principle of our profession. What is at stake is nothing less than our opportunity to succeed as we define success—as health-care professionals. Make no mistake, Wall Street and its foot soldiers, corporate dentistry, have your patients and your practice in their sights. They intend to replace you with a professional "drone" that looks and acts like you, and the public assumes—is driven by—the same altruistic service ethic we have given them good reason to trust. I think it is safe to say that Wall Street cares very little for our patients' overall dental health beyond their superficial, carefully crafted public image. And the only interest they have in you is their need to indoctrinate you as an indistinguishable, standardized, readily replaceable mannequin; you will have no control over the care their patients receive from you, when and how long you will work, or how much less they will pay you. If you have watched this as I have during my twenty-six years in solo private practice in southern California, you probably have experienced many of the same emotions—from anger to fear and frustration. Was this my destiny? Many times I have felt adrift professionally, searching for solutions that would restore my confidence in my professional future. You see, I love what I do; I love the patients I serve, and I love serving them. I want to grow in knowledge and proficiency every day that I practice—for the improved welfare of my patients, to earn an increasing reward for myself, and for the great team of professionals I am blessed to work with, who feel the same way. I want my stress level to go down as my success goes up. I found these very same beliefs present as driving principles in my friend, Dr. Mark Costes.

I have attended many business CE courses and listened to speakers in person, on tape, and via the Internet. My staff and I enthusiastically attend our state's annual scientific session. I've had no less than three different practice management consultants over my twenty-six years, each having plenty of dogma and a pearl or two that produced some gains.

The struggles remained the same. I was just surviving at a new level. My stress level had not decreased. My professional outlook was certainly no brighter—for me personally or for solo practitioners as a whole. Nothing gave me the understanding of what I was to do or the confidence that today's success would endure in the face of the impostor that is corporate dentistry. What I needed was nothing less than an epiphany.

It takes more than the usual weekend seminar to produce an effective transformation in our practices. This was certainly true in my case. What I needed was a shift in my approach—true commitment beyond merely writing a check for attendance and entrusting my future to a paid advisor. I was looking for someone who had risked their personal and professional success and had ethically achieved great results professionally and financially. I was searching for a mentor. What, or, I should say, who I found, is so much more. Dr. Mark Costes's leadership in creating a model for repeatedly building successful dental practices around solo providers is not just what I needed; it's what will ultimately strengthen the traditional dental practice business model, ensuring our ability to be the masters of our professional destiny.

Through years of dogged determination to learn, understand, experiment with, and refine a new-age application of current successful marketing and business strategies, Dr. Mark Costes shares what has repeatedly worked for him. If your efforts have brought you more than the average success but have reached a plateau, Dr. Costes shares ideas that will propel you through that stubborn invisible ceiling that has brought so much frustration. If you have had little or no success with the old standard practice management rehash and have been searching for something, or someone, to ignite the successful practice within your grasp, you will find it with Dr. Costes. What I believe you will find is nothing less than invigorating. It certainly continues to be for me every day.

Right now, you are being challenged—challenged by the winds of change—whether you choose to acknowledge them or ignore them. I invite you to open yourself up to the possibility of success that others just like you have achieved with Dr. Costes. The opportunity is real. It's right here—here and now—within the pages of this book.

CHAPTER 1:

DEFYING THE ODDS

"I will prepare, and some day
my chance will come."
—Abraham Lincoln

Whenever I speak on stage or give a presentation, I try to mention the fact that I am a first generation American. I do this simply because it is such a huge part of who I am.

It's difficult to express how grateful I am to my parents for all of the sacrifices that they have made for our family and me.

In the late 1960s, my father wasn't the typical immigrant who was fleeing political or religious persecution when he decided to leave his home country of the Philippines. In fact, he was a successful college math professor with dual bachelor's degrees in electrical and mechanical engineering as well as a master's in business administration.

His decision was especially difficult because he was newly married with a pregnant wife, and he played a very big role in supporting his parents and siblings. Because my grandfather worked for the Philippine government, he did not make enough money to support his family entirely. For that reason, my father began working as a young child to help his family in any way that he could.

Not only was my father able to help his family with the necessities, but he was also able to put two of his sisters through college and dental school.

But even though he had an incredibly close family unit, a good job, and a brand-new, pregnant wife, my father had the courage and wisdom to realize that his children and wife—as well as all future generations— would have more opportunity and a better life in the United States.

So in 1967, when my father heard about a program called "Third Preference," an American program allowing certain professionals such as engineers to immigrate to the United States, he applied and was accepted. This single, insightful decision changed the destiny of my entire family for generations.

His American dream began in Chicago, where his plane landed. Not knowing a single person in his new country, he started out with a suitcase, $150 in his pocket, and no job prospects. He rented a small room from an elderly couple and began his search for a job.

His initial goals were very simple. First, he needed to find a job so that he could save up enough money to buy a one-way plane ticket for my mother and my sister (whom he had not yet met), and second, he had to have enough money so that once the family was together, they would have their own home to live in.

It wasn't long before he phoned my mother with great news: He had hit the "jackpot." He had secured an interview with the largest and most well-known electronics company in the world, IBM. Within a couple of weeks, he was offered a job as an electrical engineer and started immediately. A few short weeks later, my mother and sister were in New York, living in their first home in America.

In 1971, I was born in Vassar Hospital in Poughkeepsie, New York.

· · ·

I'VE BEEN MOVED

Anyone who has worked for International Business Machines (IBM) knows that the inside joke of the company is that IBM actually stands for "I've Been Moved."

This joke got started because during many phases in IBM's history, the company regularly moved its employees throughout the country and the world, depending on logistical need. It was understood and accepted within the company culture that if you wanted to move your way up the corporate ladder, you could expect transfers.

As I was growing up, my family moved from New York to Colorado; from Colorado to Arizona; and from

Arizona to California—and many different towns within those states. Constantly being the new kid in class had its challenges, but the fact that I was always involved in individual and team sports helped me to make friends quickly—no matter where we ended up.

Because my father spent most of his childhood working, and because the Philippines didn't offer many options for organized youth activities, he missed out on team sports as a child. So from the time I was four years old, my parents signed me up for every individual and team sport that was offered. This turned out to be one of the best things they could have done for me.

When I was a junior in high school, my family lived in Tucson, Arizona. It had been several years since our last move, so it finally felt like we had planted roots and found a permanent home. But then my dad got the "call" once again. This time, we were being transferred to Southern California.

For any teenager, getting uprooted in the middle of high school is an earth-shattering event. Moving away from the friends that I had known since second grade was difficult, to say the least. Thankfully, my transition to a new school went relatively smoothly because, once again, I had team sports to fall back on.

As a left fielder on the baseball team, I was accustomed to playing on a field with a deep left-field fence and a warning track. During my very first varsity game at my new high school, on an unfamiliar field, I collided with the shallow left field fence while attempting to field a deep fly ball. A sports photographer from the local newspaper captured the entire scene in a gruesome three-picture sequence. Picture one showed me running full speed, face first, into the fence. Picture two showed my coach and several of my teammates on their hands and knees searching for my teeth in the left-field grass. The third pictured me being helped off the field, my jersey covered in blood.

The impact caused me to lose tooth number eight, which was never found. Tooth number nine was driven distally and rested in the middle of my palate at about the level of the second premolar. Teeth numbers seven and ten were fractured with nerve exposure, and I had an alveolar fracture from teeth numbers six to eleven. I was rushed to the hospital, where I was met by a trauma team.

When I woke up, I had dozens of stitches, tooth number eight was gone, and teeth numbers nine, six, and eleven were splinted in place with ortho wire. The fence clearly won that battle!

Even though the process of repairing my mouth and jaw was long and painful, it completely fascinated me. I actively and eagerly participated in my restorative treatment plan, made my own decisions, and asked lots of questions. I quickly gained an incredible respect and admiration for the team of dentists and dental specialists that worked together to correct the effects of the violent collision.

It's strange how misjudging the trajectory of one fly

ball in a high school baseball game completely changed the trajectory of my entire life.

From that point on, I knew what I wanted to do. I was going to be a dentist.

. . .

"I DON'T BELIEVE YOU HAVE THE APTITUDE FOR IT..."

After high school, I had a short and unsuccessful attempt at college athletics. For one year, I played football for a small school just outside Los Angeles.

The football team was assigned a small group of academic advisors whose primary goal was to make sure that all of the players remained academically eligible to play on Saturdays. During the first meeting with my advisor, she immediately handed me a piece of paper as I entered her office. This particular advisor had the reputation of having zero personality or sense of humor. The other players warned me to keep my conversation and comments to a minimum and to get out of there as soon as possible.

As I began to read what was written on the paper, I realized that it was my schedule for the upcoming semester, and that she had picked all of my classes for me. Although I'm sure she meant well, I had absolutely no interest in any of the classes that she had selected for me. When I told her that I wanted to start taking the classes that were necessary to get into dental school, she looked at me in a confused and irritated manner. I still vividly remember what she said to me next.

"Mark, do you realize how difficult it is to get into dental school? It is unbelievably competitive, and the coursework you need to take just to apply is really very tough. And based on your high school transcript, I don't believe that you have the aptitude for it. Have you ever considered a degree in recreation or physical education?"

That first meeting with my advisor really shook my confidence. Maybe I *was* deluding myself into thinking that I could get into dental school. Maybe I *didn't* have the aptitude. Maybe I should major in physical education or recreation.

That semester, I ended up taking some of the classes that my advisor had "recommended" and some of the classes that were prerequisites for the predental coursework. I struggled to maintain a decent GPA while I juggled athletic and academic demands.

As for football, well, that was another rude awakening. The gap between a high school standout and a collegiate standout was larger than I had ever imagined. The size, speed, and skill of the elite athletes at the college level blew my mind. It wasn't long before I came to the realization that I didn't have the physical gifts necessary to stand out at the collegiate level.

The writing was on the wall. After the first season—and a shoulder and back injury—I decided that it was time to move on. The following fall, I transferred to the University of California, San Diego.

• • •

NOT THE TYPICAL PRE-DENTAL STUDENT

My undergraduate experience was far from typical. Since my parents were recently retired and I was deathly afraid of debt, I felt at the time that my only option to finance my education was to work full time and pay for my tuition and expenses as I went. There were times when I had three jobs: working as a personal trainer, a bouncer at a bar, and a kick-boxing instructor—and any other odd job I could find. On top of all of that, I was active in my national fraternity and was taking a full pre-dental course load.

From a financial standpoint, I was able to graduate from UCSD completely debt-free and without taking out a single student loan. But from an academic perspective, working full time while simultaneously taking a full academic course load took its toll on my GPA.

I graduated with a BA in psychology and completed the pre-dental courses. Looking back, it seems clear that working less and focusing more on academics would have been a better decision—even if it meant taking out a few student loans. I knew that admissions committees primarily looked at three numbers: overall grade point average, science grade point average, and dental aptitude test scores. My GPA was good but not great, and my DAT scores were average.

As I filled out the dental school applications, all of the old insecurities crept back. The voice of my first academic advisor rang in my head over and over again: "Do you realize how difficult it is to get into dental school?... I don't believe you have the aptitude for it..."

I decided to apply to ten schools to increase my chances of getting an interview somewhere. Surely, if the committees just gave me a chance to tell my story, if they heard about how I worked three jobs to pay for school, how the unfortunate accident changed my life, how I couldn't picture myself doing anything else, how my GPA and DAT didn't tell the complete story....

•   •   •

ENVELOPE BAD—PACKET GOOD

Everybody I knew that had already gone through the gauntlet of the dental school application process told me that you could tell whether or not you had been accepted or rejected based on the size of the envelope that came in the mail. A regular business-sized envelope was a rejection, and a packet was either an acceptance or an interview request.

Several months after I submitted the applications, I anxiously awaited word from the ten schools that I had applied to. I envisioned conference rooms filled with committees of people sitting around big tables surrounded by stacks and stacks of applications. I figured that the stacks were arranged into three piles:

1. the "Yes" pile
2. the "No" pile, and
3. the "Maybe" pile.

I was hoping that I would somehow end up in the maybe pile and get an interview at a few of the schools I had applied to.

I wondered if these committee members had any idea how much was riding on their decisions. I was hoping and praying for the outside chance that someone on one of the panels had actually read and connected with my essay. I was banking on the possibility that there was just one committee member out there who considered life experience and hard work as important as "my big three" scores. After all, wasn't there more to being a great dentist than the ability to memorize and regurgitate information?

As the weeks went by, each trip to the mailbox was filled with anxiety. My ritual was to approach the box and chant in my head, "Packet, packet, packet, packet...." The first rejection letter I received took the wind out of my sails a bit. The voice of the academic advisor rang in my head, "Do you realize how difficult it is to get into dental school?..."

Okay, no big deal, I've got nine more chances to get an

interview. It only takes one, right?

The next two weeks were filled with disappointment after disappointment as I received letter after letter thanking me for applying but informing me once again that I didn't make the cut.

Three weeks after I received my first letter of rejection, I received my tenth—ten applications, ten rejections. I kept them all in a shoe box as some kind of sick souvenir of the whole heart-wrenching process.

· · ·

WHAT PLAN B?

I hadn't really anticipated that I would get rejected by all of the schools that I had applied to. Now that I had completed my bachelor's degree and hadn't gotten into dental school yet, I was officially in limbo. I was still working three jobs, so enough money was coming in to pay the bills, but money was very tight. I had given it a shot, and I was starting to feel like the advisor was right. Maybe I didn't have what it took to get into dental school.

So I did what every other recent grad had to do: I pounded the pavement looking for a "real" job. I went on dozens of job interviews for every position imaginable—from copier salesman to rental-car-agency representative. In two months of job searching, I got exactly zero job offers.

Apparently, graduating with a bachelor's degree in

psychology wasn't exactly the fast track onto the corporate ladder. Maybe the people interviewing me saw that my heart wasn't into it. Looking back, I'm so grateful that I never landed a "real" job. If I had, I might still be plugging away, trying to get that next promotion and hating every minute of it.

One day, while I was training a client at the gym where I worked, he asked me if I was happy with my job. I told him that I currently had three jobs, and that they were barely paying the bills. He went on to say that he worked for a catering company, and that the company was looking for someone to take over a new territory. I thanked him for the offer and told him that I had never worked in the food industry, and that the opportunity didn't really interest me. Then he told me that he was making about four hundred dollars cash per day. At that time in my life, that sounded like a lot of money! So I got the address from him and committed to show up for an interview the next day.

• • •

THE GLAMOROUS WORLD OF THE "COACH"

When we pulled up to the catering company's headquarters, my jaw dropped. The "yard" was about the size of two city blocks and was basically a parking lot for catering trucks. Back in the days when I worked as a laborer on a construction site, we called these types of trucks, "Roach

Coaches"—not catering businesses.

I vividly remember sitting in my car staring at the trucks. I couldn't believe that my life had come to this. All of the late nights and sacrifice to get my degree without help from student loans—and this was the only type of job I could land?

When I walked into the main building, I was very surprised by what I saw. The inside looked like a big-box warehouse store. It was clean and organized, and had every type of raw material that you would need to fix a gourmet meal. There were also soft drinks, snack foods, food containers, and anything else you could possibly need to operate a bona fide restaurant.

I was escorted into a back office, where I met one of the company's owners. He explained to me how his company worked. They had over fifty trucks and each had a defined territory. The company's sales representatives were responsible for getting new business and establishing the routes.

The customers were from construction sites, schools, and office complexes. The truck pulled up to the stop and blew its horn, and the customers would come out to get their food. The people who drove their trucks were not employees; they were actually franchisees of the company. The franchise owner was responsible for his or her own payroll and all expenses. Since there was a full kitchen in the back of the truck, a cook was needed. The owner could also employ a stock person and someone to clean the inside and outside of the truck.

The company generated its profit by "leasing" the territory to the franchisee and selling him or her all of the materials and supplies necessary to make the food and operate the truck. It was an extremely profitable business from the franchiser's perspective.

Since my three jobs combined didn't make half of what I could potentially earn operating the catering business, I decided to give it a shot. At the same time, I applied and got accepted to business school at the University of San Diego so that I could get my master of business administration if I were unable to get into dental school on my second attempt. For me, the MBA was a consolation prize that would hopefully open up an opportunity if dental school didn't work out.

Once again, I found myself burning the candle at both ends. I drove the "Roach Coach" from 4:00 a.m. to 1:00 p.m. Monday through Friday, and took my MBA classes from 4:00 p.m. until 9:00 p.m. every night.

It was far from glamorous work, but I couldn't believe how much I was learning about business by operating my own franchise. I was thrown in feet first without any training. I had to budget for payroll, supplies, fuel, lease payments, and maintenance before I got paid a dime. It didn't take long for me to realize that if I didn't run a tight ship, all of my revenue would evaporate with unnecessary expenses. I learned how to manage and motivate employees, balance the books, budget effectively, build rapport with customers, and make a business profitable.

Business school, on the other hand, was not at all what I expected. Most of my instructors were lifelong educators who had never actually run a successful business on their own. Most of the classes involved theory and case studies of Fortune 500 companies. Very little of the content that they were teaching was applicable to the small business owner. I began to see the whole curriculum as indoctrination into the corporate culture.

I felt like it was an ideal training ground for future CEOs and PhDs—not successful small-business owners and entrepreneurs. The ironic part of the story is that I was learning more about running a successful business by driving a catering truck than by taking MBA classes!

• • •

ROUND NUMBER TWO

Even though the experience of receiving ten rejections out of ten applications during my first application cycle was extremely demoralizing, I decided I'd give it one more try and send out a new set of applications. This time was a bit different. Instead of getting ten straight rejections, I was "wait listed" at two schools. Basically, this means that the schools had already selected their entire class, but I was on a standby list if any enrolled student decided not to attend or didn't show up for the first day of school. It was not the greatest position to be in, but at least there was a glimmer of hope.

In the meantime, I was still driving the "Roach

Coach" and refining my skills as a business owner. Within a few months, I had become one of the top franchisees, and my sales were more than twice those of the average driver. My formula for success was simple: I treated the customers like friends; I kept close track of all of my earnings and expenses; I split-tested and tracked different marketing campaigns; and I selected an excellent staff and paid them well. None of the other franchisees were operating their businesses like mine, and they were curious about my success. Since I was new to the industry, I had a fresh perspective and didn't try to copy what everyone else was doing. At the time, I had no idea how valuable this experience was going to be for me in the future.

While my business was flourishing, I was also still attending business school at night. Studying theory and case studies by PhDs who had no real business experience was starting to get old. My plan was to hang in there—just in case dental school didn't work out. I wasn't sure if it was going to do me any good, but getting an advanced degree couldn't hurt.

As the start of the new dental school semester approached, my anxiety extended beyond mailbox trips. Now my heart raced every time the telephone rang. I was instructed by the admissions offices of both schools to expect a letter or a phone call all the way up until three weeks after the first day of class. If the letter or call came, I would literally have to drop everything and leave for school that day. And I was prepared to do just that.

But the letter never came, and the phone never rang.

• • •

TIME TO MOVE ON

After two soul-crushing rounds of dental school applications, my record was pretty pathetic: eighteen straight rejections, two alternate lists, zero acceptances. It looked like this chapter of my life had finally come to a close.

I didn't want to subject myself to another year of disappointment and limbo. The dream that began seven years earlier on a baseball field in Agoura Hills, California, was over. I gave it my best shot and came up short. Apparently, the academic advisor was right when she told me that I didn't have the aptitude for dental school.

It was time to regroup and move on with my life. I got tired of the food-service business and gave up my franchise. My business took huge leaps in a short amount of time, and I was making great money, but I knew I didn't want to drive a truck for a living for the rest of my life. I continued with the MBA classes and got a "real" job as a sales representative for a wine company.

The wine company job got me out of the blue collar world and into a suit and tie. I was carrying a briefcase instead of a change dispenser. By all outside appearances, I had taken a step up. In reality, however, I was making far less money, and I was stuck squarely in the corporate structure. My boss was nice enough, but striving for her job didn't really turn me on. In fact, looking three, four, or even five rungs up the ladder in the company didn't look all that appealing either.

I went back to personal training and teaching kick-boxing to make up for my drop in income. I was working three jobs again. I plugged away and enjoyed the perks of working in the wine industry and was happy to be back in the gym training and teaching, but I knew in my heart that there was something more out there for me.

• • •

THE MAILBOX SURPRISE

One day after work, I went to check my mail. When I opened the mailbox door, mail spilled out onto the ground. There was a large package stuffed into the back of the box, causing it to overflow. When I pried it out, I looked at the return address. It was from the Marquette University School of Dentistry. This is exactly what I envisioned an acceptance package would look like, but it couldn't be an acceptance because I hadn't even applied to any dental schools for that year.

I opened the envelope, and the letter read, "Congratulations, you have been accepted into the 2002 Class at the Marquette University School of Dentistry." I wasn't sure what to make of it, but I knew that it was some kind of mistake. How could I have been accepted when I hadn't applied for that year?

I called the school, and a representative assured me that it wasn't a mistake. Apparently, several months earlier, they had sent me what I thought was an address verification form, but it was actually a supplemental application. I had actually applied for the third year in a row and hadn't even realized it. I almost dropped the phone. It had finally happened!

My new record: twenty-one applications, seventeen rejections, three alternate lists, and one acceptance! My life had changed forever.

• • •

MODELING FOR SUCCESS

For me, dental school was no walk in the park. It seemed like all of my classmates had been accepted to multiple schools and had undergraduate science majors and photographic memories. As a lifetime personal-development junkie, I had always learned that to be successful, you had to model the most successful people. In the beginning, I tried to get in study groups with the students who seemed to be doing the best in all of the preclinical classes. That strategy turned out to be a huge mistake.

The problem was that a lot of the top students didn't learn the same way that I did. Most of them came from strong science backgrounds and were previously exposed to a lot of the material that we were studying. Since I had graduated with a non-science major and had not taken many upper division science classes, I was seeing and learning most of the material for the very first time. For many of my classmates, a couple of hours of studying the night before a test was all that they needed to ace an exam. When I emulated their study habits, I struggled just to pass my classes.

It took me the whole first semester to figure out that I was modeling the wrong people. I needed to be studying with students who came from a similar background and learned more like I did. It took me awhile to realize that I would need to work harder and study longer hours than most of the people in my class—just to grasp the material. After I made this distinction, my grades improved exponentially and so did my understanding of the material.

After that first semester, I came to realize that I had to apply the work ethic that I had developed while getting my undergraduate education. I'd have to channel all of the old habits that allowed me to work three jobs, stay active in my fraternity, and take a full academic course load in the past. I was willing to do whatever it took to succeed and graduate. I didn't finish in the top 10 percent of the class. I wasn't in the bottom of the class either. I finished comfortably in the middle, which I thought was impressive, considering all of the amazingly bright people that were in my class.

Once the first two preclinical years were over and we finally got into the clinic, I felt reborn. I was finally working with my hands and on real people. We were now all starting on equal ground. Previous GPA and DAT scores and an undergraduate science background didn't matter anymore.

Now success was measured by how well you worked with your hands and how well you communicated and worked with people. What a concept!

For the first time since the start of dental school, I didn't feel like a fish out of water. I excelled during the last two years in the program. I finished all of my clinical requirements so quickly that I was able to take an externship in a real dental office for my entire senior year.

My externship opened my eyes to the reality of private practice. I was doing real dentistry at a real-world pace. I was also exposed to the business side of owning a practice. I paid close attention to the way that the office ran from a practice management perspective. I was astonished at how similar running a dental practice was to running a "Roach Coach" business—new customer acquisition, overhead control, managing employees, and customer service. There were all of the things that we were never taught in dental school.

To this day, I still consider my externship year the most valuable year of my entire dental school experience. Ironically, the biggest lessons took place outside the walls of the dental school.

After graduation, I took an associateship position with a friend of mine who had graduated from dental school three years before I did. It was another great experience. My friend and I worked well together, and I was able to further fine-tune my skills. Another added benefit was that I was also able to get an even better understanding of how to run a "dental business."

My senior year in dental school and my first year following graduation working as an associate gave me a huge head start in understanding how to run a successful and profitable private practice.

As a side note, I've employed dozens of associates in my practices over the years, and only one actually took the time to ask me anything about how to run the business side of a dental office. I've served as a clinical mentor to many, and all but one seemed to take the business side of dentistry for granted. In my experience, many dentists focus on refining their clinical skills and neglect learning about the business side of dentistry.

CHAPTER 2:

BUILDING THE FOUNDATION

"Every well-built house started in the
form of a definite purpose plus a definite
plan in the nature of a set of blueprints."
—Napoleon Hill

As a white-collar professional, my father provided a very comfortable life for my family as I was growing up. But as an immigrant and a self-made man, he was averse to debt and was always very careful with his money. So was my mother.

At a very young age, my sister and I were taught by my parents the value of a dollar and the importance of being thoughtful about every purchase that we made. We were taught to be disciplined, logical, and conservative with our money.

The lessons served me well, but as I got into my teens, I began to wonder what it would be like to be able to worry less about money and to actually enjoy spending it—rather than being terrified to part with it.

When I was about fifteen years old, I came across an old, beat-up book in my father's office titled *Think and Grow Rich*. This was the most fascinating book that I had ever read. As I explored its pages, I imagined the actual meeting when Andrew Carnegie commissioned Napoleon Hill to interview, study, and compile the secrets of the world's richest people. I couldn't read it fast enough!

Exposure to this book began my lifelong interest in personal development and peak performance. I read all of the books that I could find on the subject by authors such as Jim Rohn, Steven Covey, Brian Tracy, Zig Ziglar, Napoleon Hill, Tony Robbins, and many others. I began setting goals and did my best to apply their philosophies to my own life.

By my eighteenth birthday, I had been regularly setting goals, writing them down, and giving them a deadline—just like all of my "mentors" had suggested. By that time, I had already decided that I was going to be a dentist and had set my time frame and benchmarks to accomplish this goal. I had also set an arbitrary financial goal of becoming a millionaire by the time I was thirty-five years old.

Looking back, there was actually no good reason for the time frame or monetary level that I chose, but at that stage of my life, it sounded like a good plan.

As I mentioned in my earlier account, acceptance into dental school almost didn't happen. Fortunately, with a huge amount of persistence and luck, my life as a dental student started three years after my target date.

Graduating from dental school at thirty-one years old meant that I was about four years older than the majority of my class. A persistent feeling that I had years to "make up" dominated my psyche. I had debt from a large dental school loan, two new car loans, and a mortgage payment to cover every month.

With a mountain of debt, the financial goal that I had set all those years earlier seemed more and more unlikely. Every passing day left me feeling like I was moving in the opposite direction, even further away from my desired destination. Doubt and uncertainty dominated my mind. Rather than focus on the countless divine, unlikely, and serendipitous events that had led me to this point in my life, I chose to focus on all of the challenges and obstacles before me that seemed insurmountable.

I could have chosen to focus on everything that was right. For instance, if I had gotten into dental school on the first or even second attempt, I never would have met my beautiful wife, Leslie. By this point in our lives, she and I were blessed with two healthy sons (we now have three) who were and are the light of our lives. My parents were healthy, had moved close by, and actively participated in creating a loving and supportive environment for my boys—but I was taking it all for granted. I was blindly chasing an arbitrary goal and wasn't taking a moment to be reflective and grateful.

From my perspective, at that point in my life, I was

a mere novice in my chosen profession; I didn't possess what I considered to be superior intelligence; and I knew absolutely nothing about running a successful dental office. But if there was one advantage that I knew that I had in my favor, it was my ability to work harder than the majority of people. In the years leading up to this point, I had forged an unrelenting work ethic.

I made a conscious decision that I was going to push through to my goal—no matter how much I was going to have to sacrifice.

So I set out to learn everything that I could about becoming a successful CEO of my own dental practice. I studied, researched, and consulted with business and marketing experts inside and outside the dental profession. I applied what I could and made up the rest as I went along. I worked ridiculously long hours and withdrew from everything else. I made more mistakes in two years than most dentists make in their entire career. But with each failure—and there were a lot of them!—I did my best to adjust and correct my course.

As the years ticked by, I stuck with my plan. By now, I already had one failed partnership under my belt, but even with that setback, I kept moving forward. Eventually, even though the business was growing at breakneck speed, I started to notice that there was a major problem developing. The years at this frantic pace were starting to take their toll.

As I closed in on my thirty-fifth birthday, I felt like things were starting to spin out of control. At that time,

I was traveling between my four offices—three of which were over a ninety-minute commute from my house. I was managing a staff of over forty employees (including four associate dentists), and I was personally working over fifty hours per week at the chair. In between patients, I had to get on the phone to put out fires at the different offices.

At work, I was pleasant to the patients; but to the staff, I was cold and rigid. My stress level on any given day was usually a ten out of ten. At home, things weren't much better. My wife, who had always been my primary support system, was worried about my health and confided that she was beginning to feel like a single mother to our boys. I was missing family activities, and when I was around, I was too exhausted to be truly present.

One day, I came to the realization that the business that I had built from scratch with my own two hands was generating millions of dollars.

I had finally accomplished the financial goal that I had set as a teenager, but I was more miserable than I had ever been in my life. I had summited the mountain that I had been climbing for the last seventeen years… and I didn't feel one ounce of satisfaction or fulfillment. My blind ambition had pushed me to the successful achievement of one goal, but the journey had alienated my family, friends, and staff. Something had to change.

I decided that no amount of money was worth the time that I was missing with my family. I realized that I had become the worst version of myself, and I was in the middle of a bona fide breakdown.

As a knee-jerk reaction, I put the three practices that were the farthest away from my house on the market and sold them shortly after. Even though I was able to cash out for a huge profit, I literally left millions of dollars on the table and had potentially lost years of recurring revenue. In retrospect, I could have held onto those practices, structured the company differently by removing myself as the bottleneck, and fixed the problem quite easily. But I was far past the point where I could see anything objectively. I was looking for a quick way out of the misery that I was experiencing, and selling the practices was the only escape that I could see at the time.

• • •

WEALTH OR PURPOSE?

I am a big believer that it's not necessary to choose between wealth and personal fulfillment. You can create great wealth and make a huge difference in the world without having to sacrifice your personal values. But in order to accomplish this balance, you have to do things a lot more differently than I did.

Once again, my life has been blessed with an opportunity to do something that I am truly passionate about. As the founder of the Dental Success Institute, I have been fortunate enough to coach and mentor dentists from all over the world and help them to achieve their full potential while improving the quality of their lives and their dental practices.

As someone who was rejected twenty times before being granted entrance into this awesome profession, I am humbled to have been entrusted by so many to offer my guidance and unique perspective.

I was fortunate enough to become part of the top 1 percent of our industry, but I almost paid the ultimate price to get there. And because I have made so many mistakes along the way, I am uniquely qualified to help dentists who want to build their own empires and to do it the right way—without having to compromise what is truly important to them.

It is possible. And you don't have to choose between wealth and a magnificent personal life to get there.

I made a common mistake when I set my goals seventeen years earlier, but here's what I did right:

1. I selected a goal with a specific deadline (*the What*).

2. I identified the people with the knowledge and expertise to help me get there (*the Who*).

3. I created systems and strategies to achieve my goal by taking advice from and modeling my mentors (*the How*).

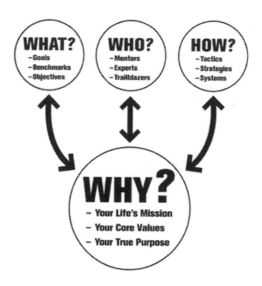

What I neglected to consider were the precise reasons that I wanted to achieve my goals (*the Why*).

Why did I want to accomplish this goal?

What was I willing to do to achieve it?

What was I not willing to do?

How could I set up my company so that it was congruent with my values and purpose?

If you fail to answer questions like these, you may find yourself right where I was—accomplishing your goal after years of hard work and sacrifice but feeling empty and unfulfilled.

Defining your "Why" provides the clear vision that you need to accomplish anything that you set out to do, without compromising your core values. Achievement of any worthwhile goal requires a great deal of planning and hard work, but as I've demonstrated by my own experience, neglecting to do the foundational work can lead to disastrous results.

• • •

PERSONAL CORE VALUES

Chapter 13 of this book details how defining the Core Values of your dental practice can help to create a cohesive team environment that has a unified set of guiding principles.

Your *Personal Core Values* are the beliefs and convictions that serve to guide your actions while reinforcing your *True Purpose*. Once clearly articulated, these values provide a framework for how to live your life.

The crisis that I experienced as I grew my own business occurred because my actions were out of alignment with my Personal Core Values. If a significant gap exists between your values and your behavior, you can never live a life of contentment, significance, and purpose.

Here is a list of my Personal Core Values:

1. *I am committed to placing my family as my first priority above anything else in my life.*

2. *I am committed to being compassionate and understanding to every person that I encounter in any capacity.*

3. *I am committed to continual improvement and striving to become the best version of myself.*

4. *I am committed to the constant positive cultivation of all of the relationships in my life.*

5. *I am committed to do everything in my power to improve the community and world that I live in.*

6. *I am committed to living a life of integrity, honesty, and humility.*

7. *I am committed to expressing gratitude for the gifts that God has given to me and to use them for the betterment of the world.*

• • •

IDENTIFYING YOUR TRUE PURPOSE

Several years ago, my two best friends died tragically and unexpectedly within eight months of each other.

I was honored when their families gave me the heart-wrenching task of delivering the eulogy at each of their funerals. In both cases, it felt like an impossible task. How could I possibly sum up everything they meant to me and how much they impacted the world in a five-minute speech? How could I possibly convey the huge difference they made in the lives of so many people?

I felt the enormous pressure of creating a worthy tribute for lives that were spectacular but far too short. I think of my friends almost every day. I now see that being able to write their eulogies was the final and most special gift that each of them gave to me. It helped me to realize what was really important to me and helped me to define my own *True Purpose*. It literally changed my life forever.

Living your *True Purpose* means that every day, you strive to become the person that you want to be at your deepest level, beyond the monetary and the material. It is the level of significance and contribution that you want to deliver to your family, your community, and the world during your time on this planet.

One of the most powerful and effective exercises for clarifying your Personal Core Values and your True Purpose is to write your own eulogy. This short speech should sum up all of your most significant contributions to your family, your community, and the world.

The following questions can be used as a guide:

- *What was your biggest contribution to your family?*

- *What was your biggest contribution to your community and the world?*

- *What did you accomplish in your life that you are the most proud of?*

- *Which values/lessons would you most like to be passed down to your family from you?*

- *What would you most like to be remembered for?*

- *Did you live a life of significance?*

The answers to these questions will help you to assemble a set of guiding principles and core values that will serve as a framework for growth and expansion that is aligned with your *True Purpose*.

With clarity in our values and purpose, decision making and planning in our personal and professional lives become much easier. With each action that we take, the simple dominant question should be, "Is this going to move me closer to or further away from my *True Purpose?*"

CHAPTER 3:

THE REALITY OF THE AVERAGE DENTIST

*"Being average means you are as close
to the bottom as you are to the top."*
— John Wooden

Depending on which survey you are referencing, the average dentist makes about $152,000 per year before taxes. If you assume that this dentist works eight hours per day, four days per week, and fifty weeks per year, here is how the compensation breaks down:

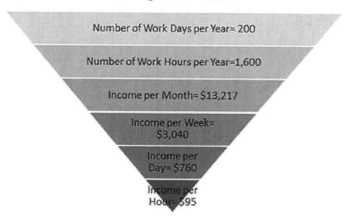

The Average General Dentist

Number of Work Days per Year= 200

Number of Work Hours per Year=1,600

Income per Month= $13,217

Income per Week= $3,040

Income per Day= $760

Income per Hour= $95

$152,000 Per year

At the time of this writing, the average American wage earner makes $42,979.61 per year. Therefore, the average general dentist in the United States is earning roughly 3.5 times more than the average American.

Upon first glance, these are pretty impressive statistics. What these numbers don't reveal, however, is the true cost that it takes to earn a dental degree.

On the average, it takes a general dentist eight years to complete his or her undergraduate and dental school education. Let's assume that the typical wage earner was working the entire eight years that you were in school. Here is how the numbers break down based on a 3.5 percent Cost of Living Adjustment (COLA) per year.

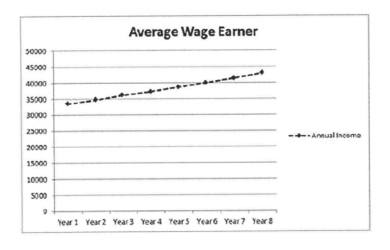

Year 8: $42,979.61

Year 7: $41,475.33

Year 6: $40,023.70

Year 5: $38,622.88

Year 4: $37,271.08

Year 3: $35,966.60

Year 2: $34,707.77

Year 1: $33,493.00

Total = $304,539.97

During the eight-year period that it took to earn your dental degree, the average wage earner generated $304,539.97 in income. But that's not the extent of his or her financial head start on you, because in addition to not having any income during those years, most dentists must utilize student loans to pay for their education. Obviously, the extent of these loans varies greatly from person to person, but based on the current cost of dental education, a conservative estimate is a total of $200,000 in student-loan debt upon graduation. If this is the case, the average wage earner has a financial advantage of **$504,539.97** over the average dentist before he or she even starts his or her new profession.

Let's take a closer look at the financial reality of a dentist earning $152,000 with a $200,000 student-loan debt, two cars, and a home mortgage.

Here's how it breaks down:

• • •

THE REALITY OF THE AVERAGE DENTAL INCOME

Income per month after taxes ($13,271 minus 30%) = $9,289.70 per month Home mortgage ($300,000) @ 5% = $1,610.46 per month

Two cars, ($20,000 each) 48 months @ 3%= $885.37 per month

Student loans ($200,000 – subsidized and unsubsidized) 20 years; average 5.5% = $1,375.77 per month

Living expenses (food, entertainment, travel, clothing, home utilities, private school tuition for children, insurance, home maintenance, etc.) =
$3,500 per month

Retirement investment account (10% gross income) = $1,371 per month

Total debt: $540,000

Total expenses: $8,747.37 per month

Total net income after expenses: ($9,289.70 – $8,747.37) = $542.33 net per month

If you analyze the expense totals in the example above, you'll see that this hypothetical dentist is not living an extravagant lifestyle. Even so, there is not much money left over at the end of the month after all expenses have been paid. You'll also notice that this does not include debt associated with purchasing or starting a dental office from scratch.

• • •

IS THE INCOME JUSTIFIED?

Although the average dentist is earning 3.5 times the national average, as the example above illustrates, there is high cost to pay to get into this earning range. Years of sacrifice and time spent away from family, the high monetary cost of education, the years invested with little or no income during your course work—this is a large investment by any standard. Then, add to the equation the challenges that dentists face on a daily basis, such as staff and management issues, liability concerns, and stress associated with patient care.

• • •

AVERAGE INCOME DOESN'T MAKE YOU AN AVERAGE DENTIST

Obtaining your dental degree means that you are part of the educational elite—not only in the United States but in the entire world. Less than 5 percent of the world's population have a doctoral degree or higher. So as a dentist, regardless of your income level, you are above average! The level of income that you achieve has nothing to do with your clinical skill, the impact that you make in your community, and the connection you have with your patients and team. But with that being said, generating less income can lead to increased financial stress, a higher incidence of career dissatisfaction, and increased work hours.

• • •

WHY DO DENTAL PRACTICES STRUGGLE?

Most dentists get thrown into business ownership without any formal business training. The traditional mind-set in the profession is that if you work hard on your clinical skills and become the best dentist that you can be, the financial side of the practice will take care of itself. This misconception could not be further from the truth. Without careful planning and the implementation of predictable business systems, any dental practice is destined to struggle—regardless of how clinically skilled the dentist may be.

Here are the top five reasons why dental practices underperform:

- Lack of effective operational systems
- Ineffective or nonexistent external marketing
- Ineffective or nonexistent internal marketing
- Inconsistent patient-retention systems
- Lack of effective systems for cash-flow and overhead control

The good news is that in most cases, income can exponentially increase, and stress and work hours can be significantly decreased with the addition of these types of systems. This book can serve as a great resource for getting any struggling practice on the right track.

CHAPTER 4:

GETTING STARTED

"Nothing in the world can take the place of Persistence. Talent will not; nothing is more common than unsuccessful men with talent. Genius will not; unrewarded genius is almost a proverb. Education will not; the world is full of educated derelicts. Persistence and determination alone are omnipotent. The slogan "Press on" has solved and will always solve the problems of the human race."
—Calvin Coolidge

It troubles me to see so many of my colleagues dissatisfied with their career choice, because dentistry has been very good to me. Aside from building six successful dental practices in a very short period of time, my other business, the Horizon Schools of Dental Assisting, has experienced meteoric growth and now has over one hundred locations throughout the United States.

I don't say this to brag. In fact, I only shared the story of my challenges and unlikely road into dentistry to prove that becoming a millionaire in dentistry is possible for anyone. And if you take the time to lay a strong foundation, you can experience a great deal of personal and financial wealth. Believe me, if a person who was rejected twenty times before getting an acceptance can do it, then so can you.

Just like my road to dental school, my journey from a young associate—hundreds of thousands of dollars in student-loan debt—to the owner of a multi-million-dollar dental business in just seven years was riddled with stumbles and huge failures.

My goal in this book is to share the tactics, strategies, and formulas that I have developed in the trenches throughout the course of my dental career. I honestly believe that the most successful business owners are not the ones who haven't made mistakes, but rather it's those who have made the most mistakes, learned quickly from them, and adjusted their course until they eventually got it right.

If you decide to take this journey with me, it's important for you to understand a few things.

1. This is *not* a magic pill

If you are looking for a quick-and-easy solution,

this is not the book for you. No true success is ever realized without real effort, commitment, and sacrifice. This is going to be hard work. I realize that there are thousands of dentists out there who are struggling in their businesses and are disenchanted with our profession. We were never taught this stuff! No one is innately born with the knowledge that it takes to run a hugely successful practice. If you trust the process, embrace the ideas that I'm about to share with you, and work hard to implement them, your dream practice and lifestyle are truly attainable.

2. You *must* open your mind

When most dentists get out of school, they are so eager to get their careers started that they focus on all the wrong things. They model what all of the other dentists in their market are doing, and they get disappointing results. Just open the yellow pages to the "Dentists" section and you'll see what I mean. The majority of the ads look identical. Everyone appears to be doing the exact same thing without any attempt to distinguish himself or herself. What I'm going to show you is the exact opposite of what most other dentists in your area are doing. This may make you feel uncomfortable, and that's a good thing! If you're willing to take a leap of faith, great things will follow.

3. You can't do this alone

The world's finest athletes, most brilliant minds, and most successful business owners all have coaches and mentors. Early on in my career, I made the decision to dedicate myself to a lifetime of learning. I've literally spent hundreds of thousands of dollars to be coached and mentored by the best marketing minds, business coaches, and personal-development gurus on the planet. I've made sacrifices both financially and in time away from my family to get to a place where I can now live the lifestyle of my choice. If trying to figure this all out on your own hasn't worked so far, follow the lead of the most successful people in the world and get a coach.

4. You *can* do this

Obtaining your dental degree has placed you in the top 2.94 percent of educated people in the United States. You have proven that you can overcome insurmountable odds to get to where you are today. You've done the hardest part! You've already made unbelievable sacrifices to get those three letters after your name. You owe it to yourself to go just a little bit further and learn what it takes to fully capitalize on your education. It's not just about the money. Money is simply a vehicle to freedom that gives you the peace of mind and flexibility to do what you want, when you want and to help as many people as you can along the way.

CHAPTER 5:

THE "ELITE PRACTICE" SYSTEMS

"To sit patiently with a yearning that
has not yet been fulfilled, and to trust
that, that fulfillment will come, is quite
possibly one of the most powerful
'magic skills' that human beings are
capable of. It has been noted by almost
every ancient wisdom tradition."
—Elizabeth Gilbert

The profession of dentistry has changed drastically in the past several years. As of this writing, there are currently sixty-five dental schools in the United States. These dental schools are graduating roughly 4,800 new dentists every year. Given the current economic climate, fewer dentists are retiring, and some are even being forced to come out of retirement due to their dwindling retirement accounts and plummeting home values. The media's bias toward reporting bad news has consumers and patients too scared to part with their money. This news has also had an effect within the dental community. Many dentists have developed a survival mind-set, retracting and waiting for "the storm to pass."

But there is some good news. There is a small percentage of private-practice owners who are experiencing unprecedented growth and success in this new economy. So, what makes these dentists so different?

1. They have an *abundance* rather than **scarcity** mind-set.

2. They have *identified and adapted* to the changes in the new marketplace.

3. They have *implemented* predictable and consistent systems that separate them from the frightened masses.

$$\bullet \quad \bullet \quad \bullet$$

THE "ELITE PRACTICE SYSTEMS"- (EPS)

During my journey from dental associate to the owner and operator of a multi-million-dollar dental company, I've been able to combine the expensive lessons that I learned in the real world with the invaluable teachings of my coaches and mentors. The end result was a series of systems that I have used to grow my busi-

ness rapidly during some of our profession's most challenging times.

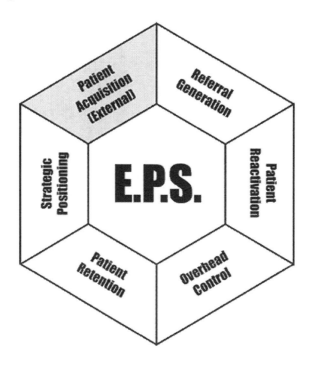

Patient Acquisition

The remainder of this book is going to focus on the
six systems that have taken me years of hard work and
hundreds of thousands of dollars in coaching and training to assemble. Mastering the following systems can
propel any dentist to the leadership position within his
or her market.

1. **Strategic Positioning** – Utilizing this system
means that you take a proactive approach to con-

trol the public's perception of you and your dental office by focusing on ways to improve your community.

2. **Referral Generation** – Patients who enter your practice through referrals cost less to acquire, more readily accept treatment, and have a higher retention rate. A practice without a strong system for referral generation has no chance to succeed in the new economy.

3. **Patient Retention** – Regardless of how many patients you are able to attract, all of your marketing efforts are wasted unless effective systems are in place for retaining the patients who come through your doors.

4. **Patient Reactivation** – Most dentists don't realize that there is a gold mine within their own inactive charts. With the correct system in place, inactive patients can be easily reactivated and create a big impact for a practice's bottom line.

5. **Patient Acquisition** (External Marketing) – New-patient recruitment/acquisition is the single biggest obstacle to having a successful and profitable dental practice. The vast majority of dental-practice marketing is costly and ineffective. A properly designed marketing piece and a

coordinated plan can create a consistent flow of quality patients into your practice.

6. **Overhead and Cash-Flow Control** – Most dental practice owners focus only on three main areas of practice performance: production, collections, and new patients. Although these are very important numbers to measure, the true health of your dental practice can only be assessed by tracking key performance indicators and comparing them to industry standards. In addition, with the correct systems in place to control overhead, a practice's maximum profitability can be realized.

CHAPTER 6:

LIFETIME VALUE OF A DENTAL PATIENT

"A great attitude does much more than turn on the lights in our worlds; it seems to magically connect us to all sorts of serendipitous opportunities that were somehow absent before the change."
—Earl Nightingale

THE LIFETIME VALUE OF A DENTAL PATIENT

Before we begin our discussion about how to strategically position your practice in the community, recruit a flood of new patients into your dental office, retain them for a lifetime, consistently generate quality referrals, reactivate inactive patients, and control the cash flow of your office, it is first necessary to define the *Lifetime Value* of a dental patient.

There is not really one agreed-upon formula within

the dental industry to calculate the *Lifetime Value* of a dental patient. The estimates range widely from under one thousand dollars to over forty thousand dollars.

All of the different methods attempt to take different variables into consideration.

In the formula below, I have used twenty years as the lifetime of a patient within a dental practice. I have very conservatively estimated that each patient will need just one major procedure every five years. Also very conservatively, I have estimated that this patient will refer only one patient to the practice in each five-year period.

The fees that I have used for my calculations are very conservative for any market throughout the United States. My goal here was to demonstrate the powerful impact that just one patient can make within a practice, even if the patient is a poor referral source who has very minimal treatment performed in a twenty-year span.

• • •

LIFETIME VALUE OF A DENTAL PATIENT

A. Five-year revenue per patient:
   a. Revenue for prophy, exams, and bitewings for one year = $250.00 or $1,250.00 for five years.
   b. One major procedure every five years = $1,000.00
   c. Total revenue per patient every five years = $1,250.00 + $1,000.00 = $2,250.00

B. Twenty-year revenue per patient = 4 x $2,250.00
   = $9,000.00
C. One referral every five years or four referrals in twenty years = 4 x $9,000.00 = $36,000.00
D. Lifetime (twenty years) value of a dental patient:
   a. Revenue from one patient = $9,000.00
   b. Revenue from four referrals = 4 x $9,000.00 = $36,000.00
   c. Total lifetime value of a dental patient = $9,000.00 + $36,000.00 = **$45,000.00**

Wow! This simple illustration demonstrates how valuable your existing patient base is and how important the Elite Practice Systems—Strategic Positioning, Patient Recruitment (external marketing), Retention, Referral Generation, Reactivation, and Overhead Control—are in building a multi-million dollar dental practice.

So here are some questions that you must ask yourself:

Are you using cutting-edge twenty-first century internal and external marketing strategies to separate yourself from the frustrated and frightened herds of other dentists out there?

Are you providing the type of patient experience that will cement your existing patients to your practice for twenty years or more?

Do you have a predictable and effective approach to obtaining referrals from your existing patient base?

Do you have a system for reactivating the patients whom you haven't seen for over a year?

Are you actively tracking and monitoring your overhead and cash flow?

If you've answered no to any of the above questions, then keep on reading, because this book will show you exactly how to maximize each of these leverage points within your practice.

CHAPTER 7:

STRATEGIC POSITIONING

"My philosophy is that not only are you
responsible for your life, but doing the best
at this moment puts you in the best place
for the next moment."
- Oprah Winfrey

Strategic Positioning – intentionally controlling the public's perception of you and your dental office by positioning yourself as an expert and trusted authority while focusing on ways to improve your community.

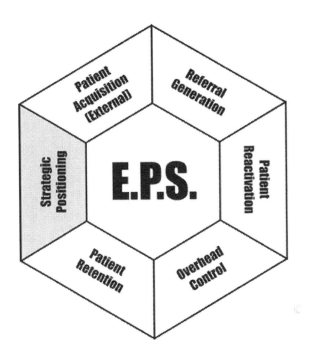

Strategic Positioning

Dentistry can be a very stressful profession. The dentist and practice owner is expected to manage and lead a team of employees and run all aspects of the associated business while simultaneously providing exceptional dental care to patients who often have unrealistic and irrational expectations.

Studies have shown that dentists as a whole have a disproportionately high level of career dissatisfaction compared to the general working public.

One of the most effective ways to combat career dissatisfaction and improve team morale is to provide more charitable dental services and to increase your involvement within your own community.

Creating a "culture of service" gives the dental team a renewed sense of purpose and pride while positioning you as a leader. "Giving back" directly helps those that you serve and creates fertile ground for growth and expansion within the practice. It is truly a win-win scenario.

The act of strategically positioning yourself can have several positive effects:

1. It will allow you to "do more good," which will improve the lives of those you touch. As a fortunate side effect, community outreach can potentially decrease burnout and will help you to regain your passion for dentistry. It is easy to forget the positive impact that we, as dentists, can have on the lives of others by utilizing our valuable skill set.

2. By proactively educating the general public as well as your patient base by answering the most frequently asked dental- health questions via print, direct mail, and newsletters (digital and physical), you can position yourself as the "go-to" expert in your community.

3. Supporting local nonprofit and charitable orga-

nizations within your community will help to expand the benefits of their good works while aligning you with them. Many of these small organizations create a positive impact on those that they serve but are seriously lacking in exposure and funding. Identifying and sponsoring these groups gives them much needed capital and exposure while giving you the goodwill created from supporting a good cause. Once again, a win-win scenario.

Strategic Positioning can effectively eliminate competition by turning you and your practice into a "category of one." This is accomplished by utilizing the following techniques.

• • •

PRESS RELEASES

Several years ago, I attended a seminar featuring a speaker with a presentation titled "How to get thousands of dollars of free publicity!" Basically, this speaker taught the audience members how to use press releases to get their businesses free advertising and publicity. The presenter covered the mechanics of creating a press release, including how to reach the contact person in charge of selecting which press releases got published and the correct format of a press release.

When I got home from the seminar, I was excited to apply all of the information that I had learned about press releases. My goal was to submit one press release to my local newspaper every two weeks until I got published. I submitted articles about the newest clinical techniques that I had learned in recent continuing education seminars, about the newest dental gadgets that I had purchased, and about the most recent certifications I had received. I did this religiously for five straight months…with exactly zero articles published.

After the five-month mark, I was frustrated and discouraged. I finally quit writing press releases and gave up on the idea of being able to get free publicity for my practice.

The most important element that the speaker neglected to discuss was the types of stories that were typically picked up and actually printed.

Several months later, just before Thanksgiving, I had a patient in my chair telling me the story of a family from her church that fell on tough times and was unable to afford Thanksgiving dinner for their family that year.

I offered to "sponsor" this family and buy their Thanksgiving dinner for them. This felt so great that my team and I decided to call several schools and churches in the area to ask if they knew of any other families in need. That year, we were able to feed over one hundred people who were not able to afford Thanksgiving dinner.

We took pictures of the team assembling the boxes full of food, which included all of the fixings for a traditional Thanksgiving meal.

After the food drive was over, it dawned on me that this type of community outreach would make a great press release. So once again, I followed the basic press-release format that I had learned at the seminar, and I submitted it to the local newspaper.

The very next day, there was an article featuring my dental office with the pictures I had submitted. For weeks following that article, we received phone calls and letters thanking us for our generosity. Some were from the actual recipients of dinners, and some were from members of the community who just wanted to say thanks for being so generous.

I'd estimate that we got at least twenty-five new patients from that single article.

Was that my intention when we organized the food drive? Absolutely not, but the unintended side effect of our community outreach taught me a valuable lesson: you can do good works and literally change lives within your community while building your patient base and improving the profile of your dental office.

The final element of the press-release strategy is that the articles that are most likely to get published are those that involve human-interest stories and giving back to the community.

Although articles regarding the latest and greatest news and advancements in the dental profession may be interesting to dentists, the majority of the population could care less—and that includes the editor in charge of what gets published in his or her newspaper.

So, if you are interested in utilizing the press release strategy to build your position and profile within your community, remember to make the stories community-focused rather than highly technical.

• • •

PRESS RELEASE TEMPLATE

COMPANY NAME

Contact: Dr. John Doe FOR IMMEDIATE RELEASE
Telephone: 555-555-1234
Cell Phone: 555-555-3456
Email: drjohn@doedental.com

TITLE/ HEADLINE OF PRESS RELEASE
(THIS SHOULD BE IN ALL CAPS)

SUBTITLE (UPPER AND LOWER CASE)

Body of Press Release Body of Press Release Body of Press Release Body of Press Release Body of Press Release Body of Press Release Body of Press Release Body of Press Release Body of Press Release Body of Press Release Body of Press Release Body of Press Release Body of Press Release Body of Press Release

Body of Press Release Body of Press Release Body of

Press Release Body of Press Release Body of Press Release Body of Press Release Body of Press Release Body of Press Release Body of Press Release Body of Press Release Body of Press Release Body of Press Release

Body of Press Release Body of Press Release Body of Press Release Body of Press Release Body of Press Release Body of Press Release Body of Press Release Body of Press Release Body of Press Release Body of Press Release Body of Press Release

Boilerplate Boilerplate Boilerplate Boilerplate Boilerplate Boilerplate Boilerplate Boilerplate Boilerplate Boilerplate Boilerplate BoilerPlate

For more information or to schedule an interview with Dr. Doe, please call 555-555-1234 or e-mail at drjohn@doedental.com.

• • •

TITLE/HEADLINE:

This states the purpose of the Press Release in the most exciting and brief manner possible.

SUBHEAD: In the subhead, you want to build up anticipation for the coming content without giving too much away. Some call this the "hook."

LEAD PARAGRAPH:

This is the Who, What, Where, When, Why, and How of the story. From this paragraph, the reader should have a complete understanding of your topic.

• • •

THE REMAINDER OF THE RELEASE:

The rest of the release serves to support the claims made in the headline, subhead, and lead paragraph. This is the appropriate place to utilize supporting material such as quotations, studies, or research.

• • •

BOILER PLATE:

This is general informational text used at the bottom of your press releases that should consist of no more than three to four sentences. It should offer general background information about a company or individual.

Example: Dr. Mark Costes is a general dentist, entrepreneur, and business coach serving the dental industry. He has launched several successful enterprises, including six dental offices, a discount dental plan, and a dental-assisting school curriculum that has been utilized in over one hundred dental offices throughout the United States.

. . .

COMMUNITY OUTREACH SPONSORSHIPS

In addition to press releases, each month our office sponsors a local nonprofit organization and donates money to its cause.

Within each marketing piece, we set aside a certain amount of "real estate" to feature our "community outreach" partner of the month. We include the organization's logo and mission statement or a brief explanation of what service the organization provides to the community.

We also feature these organizations on our website and on a special wall in the reception area of our office.

These organizations seek us out and are ecstatic to be associated with us because, in addition to the money that we donate to their cause, they receive free publicity within our marketing piece. This increases the community awareness of their good works and positions our office as a leader in the community.

Additionally, people who are already supporters of the organization that you are helping to promote will now be drawn to your office.

One particular month, we donated 100 percent of the proceeds from our new-patient exams to the canine unit of our local police department. As a result, more than half of our local police officers and their families are now patients of my office.

This type of response has occurred over and over again with many different organizations.

Once again this serves the purpose of helping the community while simultaneously building our practice.

• • •

ASK-THE-DOCTOR ARTICLES

Another strategy for strategically positioning yourself as a leader and an expert within your community is to have a recurring article or column that is published on a regular basis. This article can be written on a topic selected and researched by you or it can be the answer to a question posed by a reader or patient.

I have a weekly "Dear Dr. Mark" article that is published each month in a local newspaper. The questions that I answer are submitted to the newspaper from readers, or they are simply the most frequently asked questions that I field from my own dental patients within my practice.

Depending on your particular market, getting published in a local newspaper can be challenging. First, it's important to note that the distribution of the periodical is not important. Even if the newspaper, magazine, or mailer reaches only a limited number of people, it should still be considered as an option for publication.

The reason that you should not be overly concerned

with circulation is that the goal is to be able to repurpose the article in many different areas to maximize its impact.

For instance, you can republish the same article and feature it in a digital or physical newsletter that will go out to your existing patient base as well as prospective patients; you can also feature the article on the walls of your reception area; and it can also be highlighted within your own website.

By repurposing this one article in so many ways, the actual circulation of the original article becomes significantly less important.

As a busy practitioner, you may be asking yourself, "How am I ever going to find the time to write and research an article every single month?"

The answer to that question is one that I am going to suggest throughout the course of this book and if executed correctly, can be the biggest breakthrough in your life and your business.

The answer to that question is *delegation*.

In this particular case, if you do not have time to write an article yourself, you can delegate the task to a staff member, hire a local person who has technical writing experience, or post a job on one of the many online freelancing websites, such as Elance or UpWork. Jobs can be placed easily on these types of sites, and within minutes, you will literally begin getting quotes from independent contractors from all over the world who can help to complete your task. You will be amazed at how easy and affordable it is to hire a quality "ghost-writer" who can generate excellent articles to which you own all of the rights.

• • •

TESTIMONIALS

Patient testimonials could potentially be the most powerful tool you can utilize to position yourself favorably within your community and your practice.

Social proof builds credibility and trust faster than anything else. If a prospective patient continually sees members of his or her own community offering rave reviews for a practitioner, their level of suspicion diminishes, and they are much more likely to become new patients and proceed with your recommendations. If your state board permits it, testimonials should be included in every single marketing piece.

Even an average testimonial is more effective than anything you can say about yourself. The most effective types of testimonials come from fans raving about you and your practice and include a picture as well as the first and last name of the patient. An additional touch that adds even more credibility is to include the number of years that the patient has been with the practice.

As with recurring published articles, testimonials can be repurposed on the walls of your dental office, on your website, and in your virtual and physical newsletters.

With each new-patient packet that goes out in the

mail, our office includes three pages of single-spaced testimonials.

While we are completely aware that most people won't take the time to read through every line, many people are surprised by the number of happy patients who are willing to share their positive experiences.

This simple practice helps to set the tone for the upcoming appointment and begins building a trusting relationship before the new patient even steps foot into your office.

• • •

By utilizing press releases, community outreach sponsorships, recurring dental articles and testimonials, you can strategically position yourself as the "go-to" community leader and expert.

TESTIMONIAL AND PHOTOGRAPH RELEASE FORM

Name: _____

Address: _____

_____

What is your overall feeling about your experience
at our office? _____

_____

_____

_____

Describe in detail a specific experience with us
that you were happy with: _____

_____

_____

_____

Thank you very much!

We appreciate your honest answers.

_____ I authorize you to use my name and/
or picture in any of your promotional material(s).

Signature: _____

Date: _____

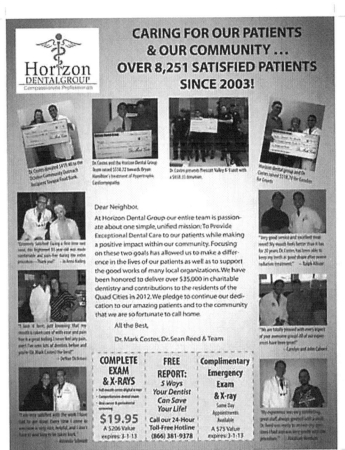

Oversized Postcard Front

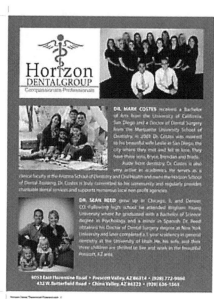

Oversized Postcard Back

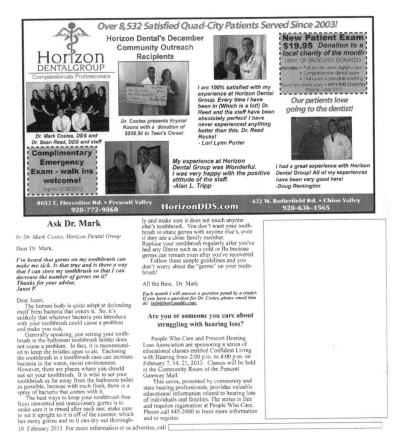

Ask Dr. Mark

by Dr. Mark Costes, Horizon Dental Group

Dear Dr. Mark,

I've heard that germs on my toothbrush can make me sick. Is that true and is there a way that I can store my toothbrush so that I can decrease the number of germs on it?
Thanks for your advise.
Janet P.

Dear Janet,

The human body is quite adept at defending itself from bacteria that enters it. So, it's unlikely that whatever bacteria you introduce with your toothbrush could cause a problem and make you sick.

Generally speaking, just setting your toothbrush in the bathroom toothbrush holder does not cause a problem. In fact, it is recommended to keep the bristles open to air. Enclosing the toothbrush in a toothbrush case can increase bacteria in the warm, moist environment. However, there are places where you should not set your toothbrush. It is wise to set your toothbrush as far away from the bathroom toilet as possible, because with each flush, there is a spray of bacteria that comes with it.

The best ways to keep your toothbrush free from unwanted and unnecessary germs is to make sure it is rinsed after each use; make sure to set it upright so it is off of the counter, which has many germs and so it can dry out thorough-ly and make sure it does not touch anyone else's toothbrush. You don't want your toothbrush to share germs with anyone else's, even if they are a close family member.

Replace your toothbrush regularly after you've had any illness such as a cold or flu because germs can remain even after you've recovered.

Follow these simple guidelines and you don't worry about the "germs" on your toothbrush!

All the Best, Dr. Mark

Each month I will answer a question posed by a reader. If you have a question for Dr. Costes, please email him at: info@horizondds.com.

Are you or someone you care about struggling with hearing loss?

People Who Care and Prescott Hearing Loss Association are sponsoring a series of educational classes entitled Confident Living with Hearing from 2:00 p.m. to 4:00 p.m. on February 7, 14, 21, 2013. Classes will be held at the Community Room of the Prescott Gateway Mall.

This series, presented by community and state hearing professionals, provides valuable educational information related to hearing loss of individuals and families. The series is free and requires registration at People Who Care. Please call 445-2480 to learn more information and to register.

10 February 2013 For more information or to advertise, call

Recurring Advice Column with Sample Ad

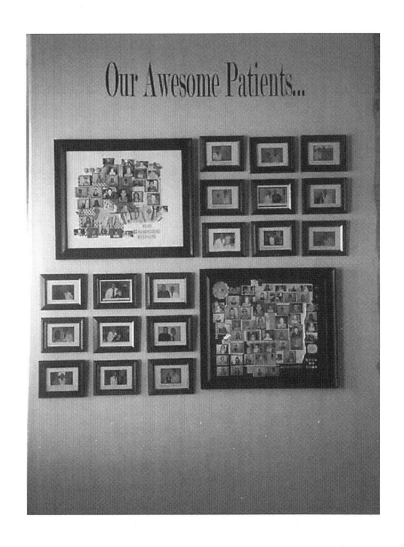

Wall of Recognition and Patient Testimonials

CHAPTER 8:

PATIENT ACQUISITION
EXTERNAL MARKETING

"I haven't failed. I've found 10,000 ways that
don't work."
—Thomas Edison

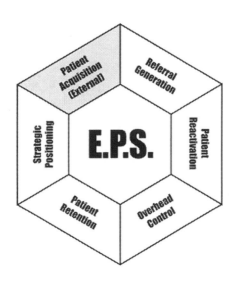

Patient Acquisition – External Marketing

One of the most critical factors to building and sustaining a multimillion-dollar dental practice is the ability to generate a steady stream of new patients who enter your practice every month.

Patients find their way into your office through two different channels: internal marketing (referrals) and external marketing (direct mail, print ads, radio, television, yellow pages, social media, search engine optimization, etc.). This chapter will focus on external marketing and how the proper design of a marketing piece and a well-planned campaign will give you a distinct advantage over the other dentists in your area.

The world of external marketing can be separated

into two distinct styles. Image advertising, also known as brand building, attempts to expose consumers to a company's name and image with enough repetition that when a product or service is needed, that company will come to mind. This type of advertising is also referred to as one-step marketing because it appeals only to consumers who are immediately ready to purchase a product or service. With this type of marketing, there is no attempt to gather a prospective customer's contact information to cultivate a relationship or follow up with the prospect.

From a small-business owner's perspective, there are several shortcomings with this type of marketing. A major problem is that the effectiveness of these types of ads is not trackable.

An example of this type of advertising is a full-page ad in a magazine featuring a celebrity holding a soft drink. The sole purpose of this type of marketing piece is to get the consumer to recognize the brand by repeated exposure in various different types of media.

There is no attempt to gather the customer's contact information, no specific instructions for the consumer, and no call to action. In this type of marketing, the "sales pitch" is implied. The ad is basically implying that purchasing this soft drink will make you more like the celebrity endorser. The company placing the ad is also hoping that any good feelings that you have for the celebrity will transfer to its product.

As you might imagine, this type of advertising may

work for billion-dollar companies with multi-million-dollar marketing budgets, but it is not at all practical for the small independent business owner.

Despite the fact that these types of ads are best avoided by dentists and other small businesses, many fall into the trap of wasting money on their own version of image advertising.

Another problem with this type of marketing is that there is very little that separates one ad from any other.

It's a phenomenon known in direct-marketing circles as "marketing incest." In our profession, this occurs when a dentist with the best of intentions sets aside a marketing budget with the goal of attracting new patients to his or her dental practice.

Since most dentists were never taught how to design an effective marketing piece, they are left taking advice from an advertising representative who knows no more about attracting quality patients than the dentist does.

The result is an ad that looks or sounds exactly like everything else out there. Most contain:

- a stock picture
- a cheesy tagline
- a list of procedures that are performed at the office
- an office address and phone number
- the doctor's credentials

I can't tell you how many times I've had frustrated dentists complain to me that they've tried marketing and it just doesn't work for them. When I ask to look at the types of marketing that they are sending out into their community, I'm not at all surprised by their lack of results.

It has been estimated that the average consumer is exposed to 850–3,000 advertising messages every day. So, a primary goal must be that the marketing piece stands out and causes the consumer to pause and take notice. Simply copying what the majority of dentists are doing or allowing the representative selling ad space to design your marketing pieces will never get you the results that you are looking for.

Now, let's discuss the alternative to one-step, image advertising: direct-response marketing.

The greatest benefit to using direct-response marketing is that it allows the business owner to capture the contact information of potential customers (patients) who aren't ready to buy at the time that they are exposed to the marketing piece. This is done by crafting and including low-barrier offers, such as free reports, twenty-four-hour toll-free messages, informational CDs/DVDs, or e-books within the advertisement. When designed correctly, this type of marketing piece gives the consumer the opportunity to move forward and purchase immediately or to take advantage of a compelling free offer in exchange for his or her contact information.

Once a "lead" is captured, the business owner can cultivate a relationship with the potential customer over a period of time until the purchase of the product or service is eventually made.

Direct-response marketing also allows the business owner to track and measure the performance of each individual promotion. This is beneficial because different elements of each advertisement (such as layout, headline, offer, body copy, etc.) can be split-tested to determine the combination that yields the best results. The dentist can then spend more money placing the most effective ads or eliminate certain types of media, dependent upon results.

For instance, two different direct mailers can be sent to two small groups of people within a certain demographic. The response to each individual piece can then be tracked and recorded. The dentist can then make an informed decision as to which ad is more effective and send out the better performer.

This process can be repeated as many times as needed to test every element of the advertisement. The caveat here, of course, is that in order to get the full benefits from direct-response marketing, the dentist has to have the discipline to actively test and track the results of each marketing effort.

• • •

DESIGNING YOUR DIRECT-RESPONSE MARKETING PIECE

Open the yellow pages to the "Dentists" section;

look at print ads that dentists are placing in your local newspaper; examine any direct mail piece that dentists are sending directly to your mailbox; listen to any dental ad on the radio....

Immediately, you'll notice a couple of things that they all have in common.

First, the majority of them are all very similar, and, second, most are utilizing a one-step marketing strategy. When you advertise in this manner, you are dealing in the "Yes" and "No" categories.

The "Yes" people have been looking for a new dentist for some time and by chance have stumbled across your advertisement. Right place, right time—they give your office a call, and you've got yourself new patients. This is obviously the desired result; but as you can see, many factors must fall into place in order to get that patient into your office.

In the second scenario, the person coming across your ad is not currently interested in finding a new dentist. He or she is in the "No" category; your marketing piece gets ignored.

So the "Yes" people have contacted your office and will become new patients. The "No" people don't call your office, and you'll never hear from them—and those are the only two options that most advertisements offer the potential patient.

But there's a third category that's neglected by almost all small-business owners. That is the "Maybe" group.

The "Maybe" group is the segment of the population who came across your ad, don't need your service right away, but realize that they might need your service in the future.

By offering a low-threshold, compelling offer designed specifically to appeal to the "Maybe" group, a small-business owner can capture a prospect's contact information and slowly, over time, establish a relationship with him or her based on education, expert positioning, and trust.

So when you're dealing in the "Yes", "No," and "Maybe" categories, your focus should be on attracting as many "Yes" people as possible but also capturing as many "Maybe" people as possible.

The "Maybe" group—also known as "leads" or "prospects"—can then be placed into a "sales funnel," which is basically an automated follow-up mechanism that could include physical letters, postcards, or newsletters as well as Internet-based follow-up instruments such as e-mail or newsletters.

The benefit of marketing to this preselected group of prospects is that they have already shown interest in what you have to offer. This makes them "prequalified" and more likely to do business with you in the future.

The most effective type of follow-up marketing doesn't necessarily have to have anything to do with sales at all. It can offer educational information or can simply be your practice newsletter that is sent out automatically.

Your goal is to stay "top of mind," and if done correctly, this group of "leads" or "prospects" will grow to know, like, and trust you. And when the time finally comes that they need your service, you'll be the only choice.

The Attributes of Direct-Response Marketing:

1. **Provides Accountability and Measurability** – This allows the dentist to track the effectiveness of each marketing piece.

2. **Makes an Offer** – This is a specific offer that compels the prospective patient to call, e-mail, or visit your website and leave contact information in return for something (free report).

3. **Gives a Call to Action** – The marketing piece will give the prospective patient an exact action to take with clear instructions (leave your name, address, phone number, and e-mail address).

4. **Utilizes Social Proof (Testimonials)** – If your state board allows it, you should always use testimonials in your marketing. Even the most poorly written testimonial is more effective than anything that you can say about yourself.

5. **Follow-Up Mechanism** – Once the new "leads" have been gathered, a deliberate and consistent process of following up is activated.

THE PATIENT ATTRACTION FORMULA

$$A + GA + P + S = QNP$$

[Avatar+ Gap Agitation +
Positioning + Solution]
= Qualified New Patient

• • •

AVATAR

Who are your ideal patients?

What are you doing to attract more of them?

You can have the slickest marketing in the world, but if you're not clear about who you are trying to attract, you'll fill your practice with the wrong types of patients or get very few patients.

Avatar is a term used among direct-response marketers that refers to your ideal customer. The more specific that you can be about who it is you are trying to attract, the better the results you will achieve.

Some questions that will help you to design your Avatar are as follows:

- Where do they live?

- How old are they?

- What are their interests?

- What organizations do they belong to?

- How much money do they make?

- What frustrates them?

- What keeps them up at night?

- What motivates them to action?

Keep in mind, there can be different Avatars for different types of marketing campaigns. For instance, sedation patients and cosmetic patients may be a different Avatar, depending on how you envision them.

Some things to consider when designing your Avatar:

• By 2017, more than 60 percent of adults in the United States will be sixty years old and older.

• This group of people will be responsible for over 70 percent of the entire nation's discretionary spending.

• So if you're marketing to a population under the age of sixty, you're speaking to a crowd that own only 30 percent of the nation's wealth.

• • •

GAP AGITATION

At its most basic level, the goal of marketing is to motivate your prospect to perform a desired action. Most often for a dental practice, this action is to pick up the phone, call your office, schedule an appointment, and actually show up for the appointment.

With the countless distractions that your prospective patients are subjected to on a daily basis, getting them to perform this simple series of actions can be a huge challenge. For this reason, your ad must elicit an emotional response strong enough to motivate the desired behavior.

Certain elements of your ad can be used to agitate the gap between the patients' current reality and where they want to be. They are as follows:

• Headline

• Body Copy

• Low-Barrier Offer (free report, e-book, video, etc.)

Headline: The purpose of the headline is to get the prospect's attention. It's literally the "ad for the ad." If the headline is ineffective, there is no chance that any prospective patients will pause long enough to look at the rest of the advertisement. Since you are trying to reach your patients in a deeply emotional way, the headline must be the area of your marketing piece that offers the greatest impact. Without a great headline, the rest of the ad will never get read.

Here are three guidelines for writing compelling headlines:

1. Identify your Avatar's most common worry or concern and agitate it.

"The Devastating Effect Dental Neglect Can Have on Your Health"

"Five Ways Your Dentist Can Save Your Life!"

2. **Ask questions that evoke emotion or curiosity from your target audience.**

Here are some examples:

"Are You Embarrassed by Your Loose, Ugly, and Uncomfortable Dentures?"

"Are You Tired of Having to Cover Your Mouth Every Time You Smile?"

"Does the Thought of Visiting the Dentist Make Your Palms Sweat and Your Heart Race?

3. **Make an indirect promise.**

"Dental Implants May Be More Affordable than You Think!"

"The Solution to Sleep Apnea without Bulky, Uncomfortable, and Expensive Machines!"

Body Copy: Once your headline has captured the attention of the audience, the body copy delivers the real message. When carefully crafted, this portion of the ad will satisfy the readers' desires and address their fears.

Most dentists fall into the trap of filling the void of the body of the ad with benign "features" of their practices. This is a mistake and is a waste of valuable real estate. The copy should enlighten the reader, create interest, and describe the benefits of visiting the practice.

In order to stay on track while writing your body copy, imagine your prospect asking these three basic questions:

1. What's in it for me?
2. Why should I care?
3. How can you prove it?

Positioning: While strategic positioning was covered in great detail in Chapter 6, its importance is worth mentioning again in this context. No matter how well your ad is designed and how elegantly the copy is written, those prospects who enter your practice in response to an external marketing piece will have some level of suspicion. Since these patients were not directed to your office from other satisfied patients, the only thing they know about you and your office is what they read in your marketing piece. Integrating elements of social proof and positioning will help to decrease a patient's apprehension and build as much trust as possible. Once the patient has physically entered your office, a well-choreographed patient experience will continue to reinforce a trusting doctor–patient–team relationship.

In addition to the benefit of building the initial trust, strategic positioning presented as photographs within an ad can be just as effective as a compelling headline in capturing the attention of your intended audience. Photographs of the doctor and the team posing with satisfied patients, presenting donations to local nonprofits, and providing community services, all serve to set your ad apart while catching the attention of your prospects.

Solution: Now that the ad has been crafted to appeal to your ideal patients, agitated the gap between where these prospects are and where they want to be, and positioned you as an authority and community leader, you must now offer a solution.

It's important to note that your *solution*, the ultimate goal of the ad, is to get the prospect in the door of your office—nothing else. It's not the job of the ad to sell dentistry—just to get them to call your office and then show up for an appointment. Once in your office, effective internal systems will educate the patient, continue to build trust and rapport, present what needs to be done, and finally complete the treatment.

Knowing the difference between one-step image advertising and direct response multi-step marketing is the first step toward realizing a perpetual, steady flow of qualified new patients. Getting out of the "marketing incest" mind-set and taking the time to design marketing pieces that stand out and allow you to capture your prospect's contact information, will separate you from the majority of competitors in your market. Following the formula above and having the courage to do things differently from the masses will give you the definitive edge.

	Date	Promotion/Referral Source	Patient's Name	Type of Exam	Result of Visit
New Patient Tracking Form				Month/Year____	
1					
2					
3					
4					
5					
6					
7					
8					
9					
10					
11					
12					

CHAPTER 9:

REFERRAL GENERATION

"Success is almost totally dependent upon drive and persistence. The extra energy required to make another effort or try another approach is the secret of winning."
—Dennis Waitley

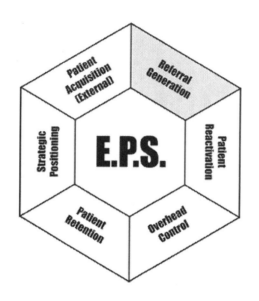

Referral Generation

Internal marketing has often been called the "lowest hanging fruit" because it can be the fastest method for injecting rapid cash into your business. This is due to the fact that patients who are referred to your office by their friends and family:

- **Possess a higher level of trust for you and your team**
- **Spend more money**
- **Stay longer**
- **Cost less to acquire**

There are many different types of patient referral-generation systems on the market today. These systems vary from simple and low-tech to extremely technical and pricey.

If you do not have some type of referral-generation system in place, then you are missing out on the most cost-effective ways to attract high-quality patients to your office.

Here are the quick and simple steps to a referral-generation campaign that I have used in all six of my dental practices. They have been extremely successful in increasing the number of new patients and office revenue.

• • •

OVERVIEW: THE REFERRAL REWARDS PROGRAM

The Referral Rewards Program is a low-tech, inexpensive system that can drastically increase the number of new patients entering your office.

This program offers a practice's existing patient base incentives for referring other people to your office. In addition to the initial incentive, the patient's name is entered into a drawing for a grand prize, which should be awarded every ninety days.

The steps are as follows:

1. Select your incentives; for best results, offer several options.

2. Select your Grand Prize.

3. Get the word out to your existing patient base.

4. Recognize your referral sources.

5. Create a "culture of referrals" within your practice.

Here is a detailed explanation of each step of the Referral Rewards Program:

• • •

STEP 1. SELECT YOUR REFERRAL REWARDS

There's not one universal incentive that works equally well across the board in every single dental office. For this reason, it may be necessary to do some testing and experimentation to determine what works best in your practice. Ideally, you're looking for something that isn't too costly from your end but will encourage participation.

Give patients a choice between three different gifts for each new patient that they refer to your office.

We currently offer the choice of a movie ticket, a large pizza, or a home teeth-whitening kit for each referral. Surprisingly, although the retail value of the teeth-whitening kit is much higher than that of the other two rewards, most patients select the movie ticket or the free pizza.

If you contact the national movie chains or develop a relationship with a local pizzeria or restaurant, you can negotiate bulk discounts.

Tip: It is estimated that up to 50 percent of people who receive a gift card or free voucher to later exchange for merchandise never redeem it. You can use this to your advantage by establishing an agreement with a local restaurant that will bill you at the end of each week or month only for the vouchers you awarded that are redeemed.

• • •

STEP 2. SELECT A GRAND PRIZE

In order for each referral source to get "credit" for his or her referral, a referral card must be filled and brought back to the office. The referral card simply has the name of the patient who was responsible for the referral. Each of these referral cards should then be placed in a clear fish bowl in a prominent place (preferably the front-desk countertop.) Every ninety days, a single card should be drawn from the fish bowl. The person whose card is drawn is the winner of the Grand Prize.

Grand Prizes should be of significant value. Good examples are big-screen TVs, iPads, Kindle e-readers, weekend vacations, etc.

• • •

STEP 3. GET THE WORD OUT

Once the incentives and Grand Prizes have been selected, it's time to announce the program to your entire active patient base. The most effective and efficient way to get the word out is by sending a letter to the active patient base outlining the rules of the program and inviting them to participate. Along with the letter, enclose several referral cards that they can hand out.

• • •

STEP 4. RECOGNIZE YOUR REFERRAL SOURCES

Recognizing your referral sources is one of the most important elements of the Referral Rewards Program.

The key to successful implementation of the Referral Rewards Program is to immediately recognize and reward your referral sources. Each referee should receive his or her incentive within two days of the referral becoming a patient of your practice. This is done by sending a thank-you note to the referral source together with referee's selected reward.

Within the text of the thank-you card, remind your patient that he or she will be entered into the Grand Prize drawing. Also, be sure to enclose additional referral cards to encourage more referrals.

The referral sources are also recognized by thanking them on a dry-erase board, which is placed in the reception area of your office. This board should be prominently displayed so that other patients can witness that other patients are participating in the program.

When designing your whiteboard, get creative!

Make sure that you delegate the whiteboard design to the team member who has the best handwriting and artistic ability.

The board in my office reads as follows: "**Horizon Dental's Referral Rewards Program**. Refer your friends or family and go to the movies or dinner on us! For each referral, receive a gift from us and have your name entered into our Grand Prize drawing!"

The next line reads, "Thank you to the following patients for your referrals!"

Then we list each patient and the new patient whom they referred. We also include a large picture of the most recent winner of the Grand Prize drawing—with the doctor and the winner's prize.

• • •

STEP 5. CREATE A CULTURE OF REFERRALS WITHIN YOUR OFFICE

Now that you know the lifetime value of a patient and the reasons why referred patients are so crucial to the growth of your practice, it is imperative that you instill a culture of referrals within your office.

The entire culture includes physical reminders placed throughout the office showing you as a team that is proficient in asking for referrals.

In our offices, our policy is that no team member will ever leave the site of a compliment without asking a patient to fill out a testimonial, take a picture with the doctor, and ask for referrals. And we get a lot of compliments because we always provide excellent customer service.

The conversation should sound something like this:

> **Mrs. Jones:** "Wow, that was the most pleasant and painless dental appointment I've ever had in my life! I've been to a lot of different dentists through the years, and you guys are the best!"

> **Horizon team:** "We're so glad you had such a good experience, Mrs. Jones! You might have noticed that Dr. Costes loves to have framed pictures of his favorite patients to decorate the walls of his office. Would you mind taking a picture with him and writing down a couple of sentences about your experience?"

> **Mrs. Jones:** "It would be my pleasure; it's the least I could do."

> **Horizon team:** "And here are a few referral cards to share with your friends and family who may be looking for a dentist. Remember, we'll send you to the movies or dinner for any patient you refer! Thanks so much for helping us to grow!"

• • •

PHYSICAL REMINDERS

Posters:

In each of our operatories and in our reception area, we have a nice framed poster with a beautiful landscape background that says the following:

To Our Patients and Friends,

Here at Horizon Dental Group, we always strive to deliver the very best state-of-the-art gentle dental care. But as you know, a world-class dental practice does not happen by accident.

We would like to sincerely thank the countless patients who have demonstrated their confidence and trust in our team by referring their friends and family to our office. We truly value each of you!

All the best,
Dr. Mark and Team

P.S. As a special thank-you, we'd like to treat you to dinner or a movie for each referral.
Ask any team member for details!

• • •

TENT CARDS:

On all of the countertops in the reception area, check-in and check-out, and in the treatment rooms, there are three-dimensional cards that say, "Refer your friends and family and go to dinner or the movies on us. Ask any team member for details!"

• • •

TEAM BUTTONS:

Each team member wears a brightly colored button that says, "Go to dinner or a movie on us— ask me how!"

By following these simple steps and making sure that all of the members of your team are actively participating in the process, your patient referrals will increase exponentially.

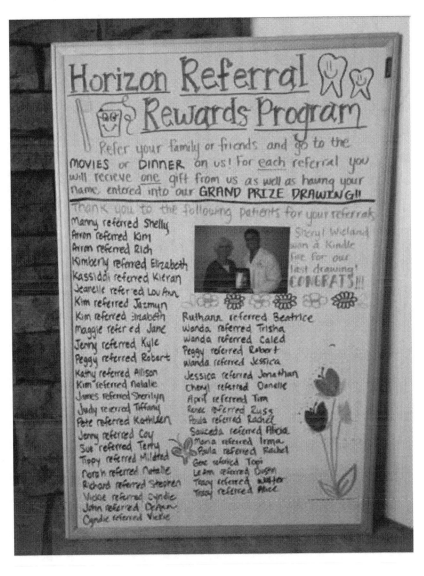

Referral Generation Whiteboard

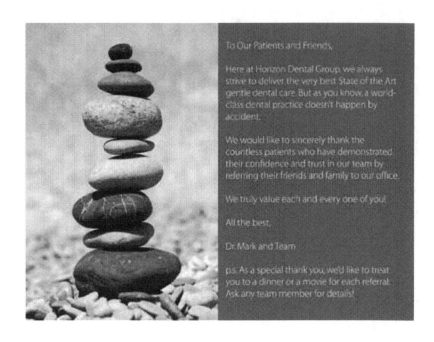

Referral Generation Poster

CHAPTER 10:

PATIENT REACTIVATION

*"Diamonds are nothing more than
chunks of coal that stuck to their jobs."*
—Malcolm S. Forbes

Most dentists do not realize that they have a "gold mine" sitting untapped in their inactive charts.

If you are currently using or have ever used physical paper charts in your practice, you know firsthand how quickly inactive charts can accumulate and create a space issue.

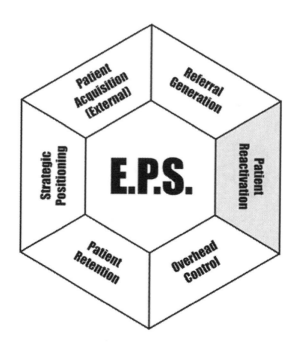

Patient Reactivation

For those of you who are completely paperless, there is less of a visual reminder, but your inactive patient list still persistently grows.

Unfortunately, once a patient has left the office and has not returned for a length of time, most dentists write that patient off as "gone forever."

What most dentists don't realize is that most of the patients who have switched to "inactive" status still live in your community and haven't sought dentistry anywhere else.

It's true that there will be some natural attrition due to

relocation, philosophical differences, and death, but most of those patients still consider you as their dentist. The majority of them just need a little nudge to get them to come back into your office and back into their healthy routine.

Dentists often send out a postcard or a letter in an attempt to reactivate patients who haven't returned to the office in some time; but if there is no response, these dentists give up and write the patient off.

It's worth taking a moment to think about why people become inactive in the first place once they have visited your office. Of course, there are countless reasons why people do not return to your practice after becoming an established patient, but let's address the most likely reasons for their absence.

1. The patient has moved away from the community.

2. The patient had a bad experience with you or a member of your team and found another dentist.

3. The patient passed away.

4. The patient has financial difficulty or switched insurance.

5. The patient likes you and your office and understands the importance of dental care but has gotten busy and hasn't been able to free up time for an appointment.

6. The patient is procrastinating because he or she is phobic and dreads dental visits.

When patients stop coming into the office without notice, it's impossible to know the reasons why. Obviously, if they are the minority and fall into the first three categories, they will never be back to your office.

The patients who fall into the last three categories, however, can be targeted for a simple reactivation campaign that will bring many of them back to the office.

The steps are as follows:

1. Use your practice management software to create a list of patients who have not been to your office for a specified period of time (for example, eighteen to twenty-four months).

2. Generate a letter offering a complimentary "Get Reacquainted Exam," including a full-mouth series of X-rays for a limited time. (The expiration date for the offer should not exceed one month.)

3. In one week, send a follow-up letter stamped "Second Notice," reminding them of the initial offer. Reinforce the importance of regular dental visits and restate the deadline.

4. One week after the second letter, send an e-mail with an attached voucher for the complimentary "Get Reacquainted Exam." Use the original ex-

piration date. If you do not have access to the patient's e-mail address, you should send a third physical letter.

5. If the patient has not responded to the three previous offers prior to the expiration date, have your team begin calling each patient, inviting the patients to the office for their complimentary exam.

Tip: If you are averse to calling patients at home, you can acquire the services of a voice broadcast company. Voice broadcast is an automated system that will call each person and a designated list and play a pre-recorded message of your voice or the voice of a team member. The message will only get played if the call is picked up by an answering machine or a voice mailbox. If a live person picks up the phone, the system automatically disconnects the call. To find a voice broadcasting company, simply do an Internet search for the term voice broadcast, and you will have dozens of companies to choose from.

Here is an example of the first letter in the campaign:

• • •

REACTIVATION CAMPAIGN LETTER#1

Dear Valued Patient,

We hope this letter finds you well. In 2012, our

team at Horizon Dental Group had the privilege of providing you with dental care. It has been at least one year since your last visit, and we are writing to say, "Hello," and to remind you that regular dental visits are an important part of maintaining your overall health. In fact, recent studies have confirmed that untreated dental disease can increase your risk of developing serious health issues, such as heart disease, heart attack, and stroke. In addition, untreated gum disease has been linked to low birth weight and diabetes.

As a reminder, regular dental insurance typically covers two exams and dental cleanings per year. If you do not have dental insurance, we are currently offering a complimentary set of X-rays and a comprehensive exam as a welcome-back gift (a value of $179).

** In order to take advantage of this offer, you must call to make an appointment within three weeks of the date on this letter. Call our office today at (928) 555-1565 to schedule your appointment.

All the best; we hope to hear from you soon!

Sincerely,
Mark Costes, DDS

REACTIVATION CAMPAIGN LETTER #2

Second Notice

Dear Valued Patient,

A few days ago, we sent you a get-reacquainted offer of a complimentary exam and X-rays for coming back to our practice.

For some reason, we haven't heard back from you. Believe me, I thoroughly understand how busy life can be and how difficult it is to carve time out of an already overbooked schedule to come in for a dental checkup. For this reason, we've decided to extend our offer for an additional week to encourage you to make that appointment.

Remember, oral health is directly connected to overall systemic health, and neglecting your smile can lead to serious dental and general health problems.

Do yourself and your family a favor and stop procrastinating!

Pick up that phone and call our office! Call our office today at (928) 555-1565 to schedule your appointment.

We all look forward to hearing from you.

All the Best,
Mark Costes, DDS

· · ·

REACTIVATION CAMPAIGN LETTER # 3

Note: This letter can be sent as a physical letter or as an e-mail.

FINAL NOTICE

Dear Valued Patient,

Two weeks ago, we wrote to invite you back to our practice with an offer for a complimentary exam and X-rays.

As a reminder, dental neglect can lead to serious overall health consequences. In most instances, a consistent routine of home care and regular dental checkups can prevent serious problems from occurring.

Untreated minor dental problems can quickly escalate into much more serious issues, which can potentially lead to systemic illnesses and tooth loss.

Call our office today at (928) 555-1565 to schedule your appointment. This offer is only valid for three more days!

We hope to hear from you soon!

All the Best,
Mark Costes, DDS

• • •

REACTIVATION CAMPAIGN VOICE BROADCAST SCRIPT

MESSAGE RECORDED BY THE DOCTOR:

"Hello, this is Dr. Costes calling from Horizon Dental Group. It's been awhile since we've seen you, and we are just calling to see how you are doing. We've sent you a couple of letters inviting you back to the practice for a free exam and X-rays. If you're interested in taking advantage of this offer, just give our office a call before January fifteenth. We hope to see you soon!"

MESSAGE RECORDED BY A TEAM MEMBER:

"Hello, this is Cheri calling from the Horizon Dental Group. Dr. Costes asked me to give you a call because it's been awhile since we've seen you here at the practice, and we'd love to see you again! Also, if you schedule before January fifteenth, we're offering a complimentary exam and full series of X-rays for our existing patients. Give us a call if you'd like to schedule an appointment. Take care!"

Utilizing this reactivation campaign exactly as its written will allow you to reconnect with the patients who are still in the area and understand the need to get their dental work completed. The key to the success of this system is following up several times. The benefit of sending two letters and an e-mail and making a phone call is that you are likely to catch the attention of the patients by using their preferred method of communication.

Reactivated patients who return to your office are similar to referred patients because they possess a higher level of trust and comfort with you and your office since they already have an established relationship with you.

Putting together a system like this and activating it at least once per year will increase revenue at very little expense to you.

CHAPTER 11:

PATIENT RETENTION

"A customer is the most important visitor
on our premises; he is not dependent on
us. We are dependent on him. He is not an
interruption in our work. He is the purpose
of it. He is not an outsider in our business.
He is part of it. We are not doing him a
favor by serving him. he is doing us a favor
by giving us an opportunity to do so."
—Mahatma Gandhi

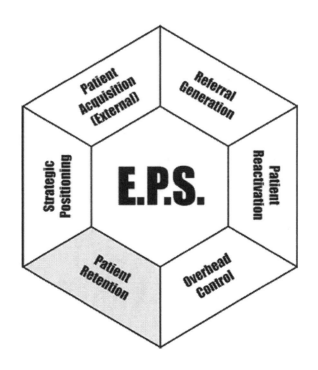

Patient Retention

• • •

THE ULTIMATE PATIENT EXPERIENCE

So far, we've covered the following: how to utilize direct-response external marketing to predictably attract new patients into your dental practice; a proven referral-generation system to obtain high-quality new patients internally through referrals from your existing patient base; and how to reactivate patients who haven't been into your practice for at least a year.

But what's equally important to consider is how to retain the potential forty-five-thousand dollar asset in your practice for a lifetime.

It's always surprising to witness how many practice owners focus their energy, time, and money on new-patient acquisition while devoting almost no thought and attention to retaining these patients.

In today's ultra-competitive environment, patients are constantly bombarded with marketing messages and low-price offers. Without a unified team philosophy, strategy, and culture, patients will literally walk in your front door and right out the back door.

The ability to retain patients goes far beyond just being friendly and polite. In order to create relationships that are strong enough to withstand all of the distractions of the new economy, each team member—from the sterilization technician to the doctors—must have a crystal clear understanding of his or her role in creating an unforgettable patient experience.

There are eight definitive stages that you must master in order to deliver a patient experience that will keep patients with you for a lifetime. Each of these stages must be handled consistently—with finesse and purpose. A structure and a script for each stage is a helpful tool, but each team member must become comfortable enough in his or her delivery to avoid appearing artificial and robotic.

The only way for this comfort level to be established is through practice, practice, and more practice. Here are the eight steps to the ultimate patient experience:

1. **The Initial Patient Call** – Answering the telephone in the dental practice is one of the most important elements for maximum practice growth and patient retention. The results of the internal and external marketing efforts are dependent upon how well the front desk team handles new patient calls. Rapport and relationship building begin at this call, and its importance is paramount.

Key points to mastering the initial phone call:

a. Lower the barriers

All team members answering the phone must understand that it is not their role to qualify or filter the patients who are calling to schedule an appointment at your office. Barriers of entry into your practice should be minimized or eliminated. Each team member must be aware that the number one goal of the initial phone call is to schedule the appointment.

b. Answer the call within three rings

There should be at least one or two primary front-office team members who are the most skilled at answering the phones. However, every team member within the practice must be able to competently answer the phone in the event that the primary front-desk team member is busy with other patients. The "three-ring rule" simply means that each person within the office commits to work together in order to make sure that the phone is always answered within three rings.

c. Build rapport

Regardless of what may be happening within the dental office, when the phone rings, the team member must answer the call in the friendliest and most helpful manner possible. As early as possible in the conversation, the team member should get the potential patient's first name and address the caller by name for the remainder of the call. Being polite and respectful must be an absolute non-negotiable requirement for anyone answering the phone.

d. Categorize (don't qualify) the caller

There are six main caller categories, and they are listed below in order of importance:

New Patient – These callers are first priority, and every attempt should be made to get them into the office for an appointment.

Existing Patient (scheduling an appointment) – These callers are also high priority and should be scheduled as soon as possible. Make sure to address the patients by name and welcome them warmly back to the practice.

Existing Patient (billing/insurance question) – These callers are high priority and must be delivered the highest level of customer service. If it is possible, these patients should be referred to the billing department in order to help them get the most accurate answers to their questions and to free up the front-office team to handle incoming calls. The best scenario is to make sure that the patient has had a return call the same day or early the following day.

Vendors – These callers should be referred to an office manager or team member in charge of ordering. You must get them off the phone as quickly and as courteously as possible and have the appropriate team member return the call when it's convenient.

Personal Calls – These calls are low priority. A policy should be enacted that prohibits personal calls during business hours with the exception of emergencies.

<u>Sales Calls</u> – These are the absolute lowest priority calls. The absolute minimal amount of phone time must be given to these types of calls.

<u>Miscellaneous Calls</u> – These are any calls that do not directly fit into the categories listed above. In most cases, these types of calls should be delegated to the appropriate team member when possible.

The manner in which your team answers the telephone and handles the different categories of callers could be the single most important task in the success and growth of your dental practice. It is therefore of the utmost importance to make sure that the staff is well trained and prepared to take on the task. Neglecting this important step could potentially mean the difference between a wildly successful practice and one that struggles to survive.

2. **The Confirmation Call** – This brief interaction is important because it is the last interaction that the team will have prior to the first in-person visit to the office. This conversation should be quick and to the point, but it should also set the tone for the upcoming visit. The team member must have an upbeat, friendly, and helpful demeanor. Remember, we are inviting the prospect to join the practice.

3. **The Welcome Packet** – Even if you have a paperless practice, one of the most effective ways to build a level of trust and rapport is through an effective welcome packet. In addition to the traditional intake forms, insurance forms, and financial forms, you should include a personalized letter to welcome the patient to the practice. A letter that has a picture of the team or is personally signed by each member of the team will set it apart from the usual cold and sterile medical or dental packet.

   The most important element of your entire welcome packet, however, is the testimonials. In our office, together with all of the items listed above, we include three pages of single-spaced testimonials from our raving fans. Although we are aware that most people won't take the time to read all of the testimonials enclosed, this unexpected social proof will help to position us as a trusted community leader.

4. **Front-Desk Greeting** – Here it is—this is the first physical interaction with the new patient. Remember, you must treat this visit as if it's a job interview or audition. You are trying to get hired as his or her dental office for life!
   So far, you have separated your practice from

99 percent of all other practices by answering the initial phone call in a friendly and professional manner.

Then you send the patient a unique welcome packet, including a welcome letter and a stack of glowing patient testimonials.

Now it's time to further impress the patient with the care you show him or her inside the office.

No matter what is happening at the office when the patient arrives, all team members in the area must greet the patient with a "Hello" and a smile. Under no circumstances should a patient walk up to the front-office area without being greeted. Patients have unfortunately become accustomed to walking into a cold and sterile medical setting and signing in on a clipboard while basically getting ignored by the staff on hand. The more you can differentiate your practice from the stereotypical dental setting, the longer and stronger your relationship will be with the patient.

Any team member in the immediate area of the front desk when a patient arrives must pause and greet the incoming patient. If the front-office team members are on the phone when a patient arrives, they can smile and wave to the patient, acknowledging his or her arrival. If another team member is close by and has noticed that the patient has not received a proper greeting because the primary front-office team member is on the telephone, the backup team member must welcome the patient and begin the check-in process. Once the primary front-office team member is available, it is appropriate to hand over the duties back to the front office.

Remember: Every step in the patient experience is another opportunity to provide exceptional and memorable customer service and to distinguish you and your practice from the rest of the practitioners in your market.

5. **Transition from Reception Area to Treatment Room** – This brief interaction is an important transition that most medical and dental offices overlook. It must become part of your practice's culture that every patient is received like an old friend—with a smile and a warm greeting. This transition is especially important because the patient is getting his or her first glimpse at the back-office team. The tone for the entire team-patient relationship can be guided by this initial impression.

The back-office team member must take a quick pause and internally ask the following questions prior to calling the patient back to the treatment room:

• How do I pronounce this patient's name? (If you are unsure, verify with the front office team members.)

- Is this a new or existing patient? (Check the patient record to verify this.)

- How should I address this patient? (As a rule of thumb, our office addresses patients over fifty-five years old as Mr., Ms., Dr., etc.)

6. **Seating the Patient in the Treatment Room** – This is one of the most important steps in the entire new-patient experience. The patient is finally in the chair and is evaluating every aspect of the office.

   So far, the patient should have experienced exceptional service on the telephone while making the initial appointment. He or she was then sent a welcome packet with pages of glowing testimonials from your biggest fans. When the patient arrived at the front-desk area, he or she was greeted like an old friend and given a new-patient gift. The back-office team member warmly greeted him or her and escorted the new patient back to the treatment room.

   Up until this point, each interaction was carefully guided, scripted, and choreographed.

   This phase of the patient experience requires a bit more skill and personality. The team member must be able to have a conversation with the patient. The goal is to extract as much personal information from the patient as possible without making it feel like an inquisition. It is at this phase of the patient experience that rapport is built and the foundation for a lifetime relationship begins.

Once the patient is seated in the chair, the back-office team member should start to get to know the patient. He or she should not immediately begin talking about dentistry and what's going to happen during the appointment. We use a form called the "yellow sheet," which helps guide the team member toward the types of facts that we like to know about each patient. Each bit of information that we are able to gather from the patient allows the team to provide better service and care to the patient.

Creating an engaging conversation is an art and a skill that must be developed. Here are some quick pointers:

Have a three-question rule. At our practices, as a rule of thumb, anyone working in the back office interacting with the patients tries his or her best to ask three non-dental questions in an attempt to get to know the patient better.

Get the patient to talk about himself or herself. Studies have shown that if you direct a conversation toward people and get them talking about themselves, they will walk away from the conversation feeling better about you.

Ask open-ended questions. Ask the type of

questions that require more than a *yes* or *no* answer.

Genuinely listen. One of the greatest aspects of dentistry as a profession is getting to know so many people with diverse backgrounds and stories. Listen to what the patients have to say and develop a genuine care and interest in them. After all, we treat the whole person—not just the mouth!

7. **Introduction to the Doctor** – Once the FMX for a comprehensive-exam patient or the PA for the emergency patient has been taken and the back-office team member has had sufficient time to get to know the patient, the doctor should be called into the treatment room.

Prior to entering the treatment room, there should be a "hallway briefing" between the back-office team member and the doctor. During this briefing, the back-office team member should inform the doctor of the patient's chief complaint or reason for visiting the office, any significant medical history, and something personal about the patient.

When the doctor enters the room and begins the interaction, he or she should also follow the "three-question rule" and ask three non-dental personal questions prior to talking about dentistry.

8. **Transition from Treatment Room to Front Office** – Following the new-patient exam and the presentation of the treatment plan, the next step is to escort the patient back to the front-office team member for check-out and reappointment.

   The back-office team member must "hand off" the patient to the front-office team member. The patient should never be left alone to wait for a front-office team member to help him or her.

   By following these eight defined steps in the Ultimate Patient Experience, customer service will no longer be left to chance. By defining the parameters and expectations of each stage of this system with the team members, it gives them accountability and structure to produce predictable and exceptional service.

· · ·

PATIENT RECOGNITION

Let's face it. Most people are not recognized nearly as much as they should be. They may feel underappreciated by their spouse, by their kids, by their coworkers, by their boss, by their friends, by everyone in their lives. Yet being recognized and appreciated is one of the most basic human needs.

The reasoning behind our "three-question rule" and our "yellow sheets" is to get to know our patients on a deeper level. If they open up to the team or the doctors about important milestones or events in their lives, we always try to capture those comments on our yellow sheets.

We are constantly looking for reasons to acknowledge, recognize, and appreciate our patients. Our goal is to reach out to our patients between twelve and seventeen times per year.

We are able to accomplish this by recognizing:

- Birthdays
- Anniversaries
- Graduations
- Retirements
- Births of children and grandchildren
- Passing of loved ones
- Major milestones or accomplishments

The main vehicles for this recognition are our print and e-mail newsletters and greeting cards. Each month, we restock our card drawer with an assortment of greeting cards for all occasions. Whenever a special occasion is brought up in conversation, the team member who wrote it in the yellow sheet also writes a reminder for a recognition card and hands it off to the team member designated to send out the greeting cards for the month. The card is then filled out and sent the day that it was written out.

Birthday acknowledgment. If your office does not have a system in place to acknowledge each patient's birthday, you are missing a big opportunity. The majority of people in the world, regardless of their religious or cultural affiliation, celebrate birthdays. A simple and inexpensive gesture—like sending a personalized card along with a simple gift—demonstrates to your patients that your team cares.

In order to ensure that the system runs smoothly, delegate the tasks of this system to one or two team members. If too many people get involved, the whole process becomes unnecessarily cumbersome and inefficient.

Here are steps to the patient birthday system:

1. Create a customized birthday card, preferably with a picture of your team and your practice logo.

2. Use your practice management software to pull a report, listing the birthdays for the upcoming month.

3. The card should be handwritten and signed by each member of the team. It is tempting to use a pre-written card and a pre-signed card in an attempt to save time and effort. Do not do this. A handwritten and personally signed card stands out, and patients will take notice. In order to keep costs down, I hire a high school student with excellent handwriting to write out each birthday card. The cards are then sent back to the offices, where each team member signs them in different colored ink.

4. Establish a relationship with a local restaurant that will offer to give a free dessert to each one of your patients on their birthday. Most restaurant owners are happy to offer a coupon or voucher for a free dessert to your patients on their birthday for several reasons: For one, it is a low-cost way to increase their exposure to a large number of people (your patient base). Secondly, they realize that people typically don't dine alone on their birthday, and if they come in to redeem their dessert coupon with only one other person, both will probably buy dinner and drinks. This scenario will easily pay for the investment of a free dessert, and it will increase the patient's goodwill toward you and your practice.

5. Enclose the free-dessert coupon in the envelope along with the card. The birthday card that we give out to our patients has the following handwritten message inside:

Dear Sarah,

On behalf of our entire team, we just wanted to wish you all the best on your special day! We've enclosed a little gift for you to enjoy. Have a great birthday!

Dr. Mark and Team

The entire team then signs the card in multicolored pens to make it look more festive.

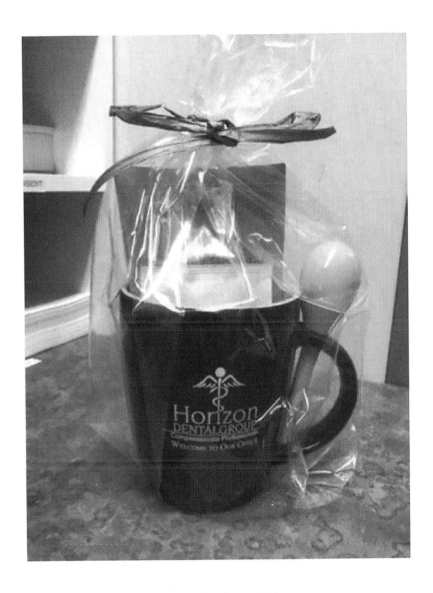

New-Patient Gift

**Dr. Mark Costes
and Family**

Welcome to
Horizon
Dental Group!

**Dr. Sean Reed
and Family**

Dear Valued Patient,

Drs. Mark Costes, Sean Reed and team would like to take this opportunity to welcome you to Horizon Dental Group. We are excited about the opportunity to meet all of your oral care needs. At Horizon Dental Group we strive to provide the highest quality dental care in a relaxed and comfortable environment. It is our goal to create life long doctor-patient relationships by delivering compassionate dental care and exceptional customer service.

Please fill out all of the enclosed forms and present them to our front desk team members upon arrival for your appointment. We look forward to meeting you!

Sincerely,

[signature]

[signature]

Mark Costes, DDS
Sean Reed, DDS

Welcome Letter

Dear Sarah,

On behalf of our entire team, we just wanted to wish you all the BEST on your special day! We've enclosed a little gift for you to enjoy. Have a GREAT DAY! ☺

LouAnne   Dr. Reed   Shelly
Devon   Happy Birthday!   Kelcie
Darla   Dr. Mark Costes   Holly
Jessica   and   Julie
SUZY   Jean   Kristie   Amanda

Handwritten Birthday Card

CHAPTER 12:

OVERHEAD CONTROL

"What's measured, improves."
—Peter F. Drucker

WHAT ARE KEY INDICATORS?

Recently, when reviewing my portfolio, my financial advisor determined that I was under-insured, and that I needed to obtain an additional life insurance policy. I decided to follow his advice and began the process by contacting the insurance company to set up the required physical exam. Shortly after, I was contacted by a traveling nurse who arranged an appointment to visit my home and perform the exam. Upon arrival, she wheeled a small travel suitcase into my dining room, where she immediately began assembling a small makeshift medical office.

The physical consisted of all of the routine tests and measurements, including height, weight, blood pressure, and pulse rate. She drew blood, which would later be analyzed for cholesterol, blood sugar, triglycerides, nicotine, marijuana, and blood-borne diseases such as HIV and hepatitis C.

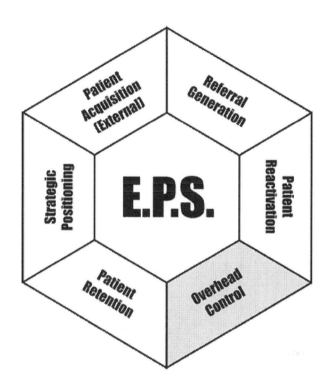

Overhead Control

She took a urine sample to be sent into the lab to check protein, glucose, and creatinine.

She also performed an EKG to make sure that the electrical activity of my heart was normal. A few weeks later, I received the test results, and everything turned out to be within the normal range. After the insurance company received and analyzed my reports, it contacted me to tell me what my insurance premiums would be, based on my "numbers."

The "numbers" were simply a combination of lab values and physical data gathered from my exam. An incomplete group of numbers wouldn't have given the insurance company sufficient information to assess my overall health (and my likelihood of dying within a certain period of time). It's clear that the insurance companies have perfected the practice of using a handful of "key indicators" to predict the likelihood of a premature claim. So, what does this have to do with your dental practice?

• • •

THE HEALTH OF YOUR PRACTICE

Dentists can learn a lot from life insurance companies. The nurse didn't come to my house, take my height, weight, and blood pressure, and leave. She performed a thorough exam to get a true picture of my health.

Many dentists focus on only three numbers—production, collections, and new patients—and try to evaluate their practices based on this limited information.

Although it is not a living and breathing thing, a dental practice also has certain key indicators that can be used to assess its health. These categories must be measured and recorded on a regular basis. Consistently committing to this practice will allow you to do the following four things:

1. **Identify the areas where you may be bleeding cash** – If a certain expense or revenue category is significantly skewed in comparison to industry standards, you must investigate and deal with the problem appropriately.

2. **Promote growth** – As Peter Drucker said, "What's measured, improves." Therefore, becoming familiar with the critical numbers that make up your overhead and revenue will allow you to correct and adjust wherever necessary.

3. **Increase profitability** – Tracking revenue and expenses allows you to control expenses and set benchmarks for production and collections. Profitability increases significantly when controls are placed on both the money coming in and the money going out.

4. **Decrease stress** – Dealing with personal and practice finances can be stressful when a dentist does not take an active role in understanding the flow of cash through the business. Simply identifying the problem usually leads to relief. Taking actionable steps to correct the problem will diminish stress even further.

· · ·

PRODUCTION/COLLECTIONS RATIO (PERCENTAGE)

There is no doubt that production and collections are the two numbers that the majority of dentists follow on a daily basis. Although production is a very important number, if your practice's production/collection ratios are significantly skewed, your practice will have no chance of realizing its true profit potential. A healthy practice will have a collections percentage of at least 98 percent of gross production on any given month. Dropping below this level will cause the accounts receivables to rise to unacceptable levels.

· · ·

ACCOUNTS RECEIVABLES (A/R)

Total A/R beyond 100 percent of a single month's production is indicative of a problem somewhere in your financial arrangements or collection protocol.

The following steps will help to keep A/R under control:

1. Develop a written financial policy that is understood by every team member and explained to each patient when the treatment plan is presented.

2. Create a documented follow-up system that deals

with insurance companies that have delayed payment, requested further information, or denied a claim.

3. Develop scripts for the team that address various financial arrangements that will be available to the patients.

4. Utilize patient financing companies and avoid internal financing whenever possible.

5. Assign "past-due" accounts to a team member for follow-up.

Key Industry Standards

Key Indicators	Percentage of Collections
Employee payroll	25% – 30%
Dental supplies	5% – 7%
Lab fees	8% – 10%
Facility costs	6% – 9%
Marketing	2% – 5%
Total expenses	55% – 65%

• • •

GETTING THE TEAM ON BOARD

Another crucial element to successfully controlling practice overhead is to create team accountability. Obviously, the first step in this process is to get a firm grasp of your practice numbers in comparison to industry standards.

Once this baseline has been established, each department should be held accountable for certain key categories. Here are some examples of departmental accountability:

Back-Office Budget:
- Lab fees under 10%
- Dental supplies under 7%
- Production above $100K
- (Numbers may vary depending on practice)

Treatment Coordinator:
- Treatment plan acceptance above 70%

Front Office:
- Number of new patients: 55
- (Numbers may vary depending on practice)

Hygiene Department:
- Production of 3x total hourly pay for Hygienist plus Hygiene Assistant

Billing Department:
- Collections above 98% of gross production
- A/R Total= no more than one full month's collections
- 60–90 day A/R no more than 20% of total

Once the parameters for team accountability are clearly defined, benchmarks can be reviewed at regularly scheduled meetings. Any bonus structure that is put in place should be dependent upon every department's accomplishing its goals and as a percentage of profit only. If the owner of the practice is not profiting at the end of each month nobody on the team should be receiving a bonus.

• • •

PROFIT AND LOSS REPORT (P&L)

The Profit and Loss Statement, also known as the

Income Statement is a useful tool for understanding the financial health of your practice. This report serves as a progress report that reveals how your practice is doing within a particular period of time. The P&L can be prepared and reviewed for any length of time but is most helpful when utilized monthly.

Revenue (total collections) for the defined period of time is placed at the top of the statement. This figure can be expressed as an office total or categorized based on the producer. (For Example: Hygienist#1, Doctor #1, Hygienist # 2, Doctor # 2)

Below the Revenue, **Direct Expenses** are itemized. These expenses include the materials, laboratory and labor costs (doctors, hygienists and assistants) directly related to the delivery of dental services.

Indirect Expenses can be defined as any expenses that are necessary to run the dental practice but not directly related to the delivery of dental services.

Net Profit is defined as the total collections minus the sum of the direct and indirect expenses.

WHERE'S ALL THE MONEY?

Early in my journey into dental practice ownership, from all outside appearances, the business looked like the model of success. Our new patient flow was strong, our production was increasing every month, and we were collecting about 98% of the associated fees from the dentistry that we produced.

But behind the scenes, there was a large problem brewing. No matter how much our revenue increased every month, the cash in the bank always seemed to run out before we could pay all of our vendors and our payroll. On several occasions, I had to dip into my personal savings just to keep the business running.

I looked to my CPA for answers. He responded by printing out a series of expense reports as well as profit and loss statements and bank account records. The reports consisted of pages upon pages of uncategorized individual expenses. I leafed through the reports not really knowing what I was looking for. I knew that the answers to all of my questions as well as the clues that would solve my cash flow dilemma were within the pages of those reports. However, from my perspective, the problem was the information that was given to me was in a format better suited for a bookkeeper or accountant. In other words—it looked like a foreign language to me!

I didn't have the time or energy to do the forensic accounting necessary to uncover the "holes in my bucket." I confided to my accountant that I would love a simpler report that contained all of the information that I needed to assess the health of my practice—on a single page. He politely explained that he didn't possess the time, expertise, or dental knowledge to create such a report.

Eventually I got better at reading expense reports and profit and loss statements, but my process was still clunky and time-consuming.

FROM FRUSTRATION TO CLARITY

One night at a cocktail party I was introduced to Jake Conway through a mutual friend. Casual conversation led to a discussion about what each of us did for a living. Jake worked as an analyst for a large hotel chain, and he explained that his role at the company was working with teams of other analysts and consultants to minimize overhead and maximize profitability of each resort in the company. The teams would gather the raw overhead and expense data, categorize it, and compare each category with the defined industry standards. Once the analysis was complete, the teams would report back to an executive team to discuss the strengths and weaknesses of each location. If corrective action was necessary, a strategic plan was created and implemented.

As I listened carefully, I began to ask more and more specific questions about their methods for gathering information and the format of their reports. In response, Jake seemed curious as to why a dentist would be so interested in the details of his job. I told him about my thriving practices and the challenges that I had faced with the tracking and deciphering of overhead and profitability. Then I explained to him that the many dentists who were my coaching clients were also experiencing the same problems. I went on to share with him my frustration with traditional expense reports and that I had been looking for a simple way to integrate a categorized expense report that would show profitability, overhead, and comparisons with the professional standards for each category—all on one page.

That night, we took elements from the reports that Jake was familiar using in the hospitality industry and simplified the reports that I was getting from my CPA. Then we drew out the first version of *Custom Practice Analytics* on the back of a cocktail napkin.

Shortly after that evening, I began using the *Custom Practice Analytics* reports in my own dental offices. Now, I also use them to track expenses, overhead, and profitability in the offices of my dental practice clients from all over the world. Our reports are constantly evolving, with the overall goal of providing the owner of any dental practice the format necessary to get a true sense of the health of their dental practice at a glance, in a matter of seconds.

WHAT'S YOUR SCORE?

Keeping a scorecard is a very quick and easy way to track the overhead, profitability, and expenses per category in a dental practice. With our system, points are given for percentage points above the target in each expense category. Negative points are given if the expense per category is below the target percentage. Once all of the raw data is compiled and entered into the report, the total number of points is tallied—the lower the overall number, the better the score.

Here is a breakdown of our scoring scale:

Less than Zero = "Cruise Control" (Excellent)
0 – 2.6 = "Ahead of the Game" (Good)
2.61 – 4.59 = "Getting By" (Satisfactory)
4.6 – 6.0 = "Needs Improvement" (Unsatisfactory
Greater than 6.1 = "Out of Control" (Urgent Intervention Needed)

In analyzing the practice "Scorecard" below, you will see how Dr. Jones' example practice measures up in each of the "Key Performance" categories for the month of September. Note: *The categories are represented as a percentage of total collections.*

September

September Practice Scorecard

Dr. Jones

Revenue (collection) $142,388

Total Expenses Excluding Dr: $98,538

Overhead % Excluding Dr: 69%

Variance of Overhead % to target of: 60% 9%

Expense Breakdown	Total Expense	Expense %	Industry Standard	Variance %	Points
Staff Salaries	$30,841.667	21.66%	16.00%	5.66%	5.66
Hygiene Salaries	$9,559.02	6.71%	9.00%	-2.29%	-2.29
Payroll Taxes & Fees	$4,593.74	3.23%	2.50%	0.73%	0.73
Fringe Benefits	$2,991.75	2.10%	2.50%	-0.40%	-0.40
Total Payroll	$46,810.93	32.88%	30.00%	2.88%	2.88
Lab Fees	$16,501.89	11.59%	9.00%	2.59%	2.59
Dental Supplies	$9,675.01	6.79%	5.00%	1.79%	1.79
Doctor Salaries	$42,454.80	29.82%	30.00%	-0.18%	No points
Advertising	$1.763.84	1.24%	4.50%	-3.26%	-3.26
Other minor	$439.47	0.31%	2.00%	-1.69%	-1.69
Other expense	$9,436.84	6.63%	5.50%	1.13%	1.13
Insurance	$2,416.61	1.70%	1.50%	0.20%	0.20
Legal & Accounting	$1,034.00	0.73%	1.50%	-0.77%	-0.77
Office Expenses	$3,044.21	2.14%	1.20%	0.94	0.94
Facility & Equipment	$7,989.71	5.61%	9.00%	-3.39%	-3.39
Telephone	$1,085.12	0.76%	0.80%	-0.04%	-0.04

Net Production vs last year	September		Points Scorecard Key	5.37
Prior Year Production	$101,775.00		<0 = Cruise control	
Current Year Production	$129,807.60		0 - 2.6 = Ahead of the game	
Variance (+/-)	28%		2.61 - 4.59 = Getting by	
			4.6 - 6.0 = Needs improvement	
			> 6.0 = Out of control	

PRACTICE SCORECARD FOR DR. JONES' (EXAMPLE) PRACTICE:

- **Staff Salaries**: This practice is allocating 21.66% of total collections to Staff Salaries. This is above the target of 16% by 5.66%. This results in a score of +5.66 for this line item.

- **Hygiene Salaries**: This practice is allocating 6.71% of its total collections to Dental Hygienist salaries. This is below the target of 9% by 2.29%, resulting in a score of −2.29 for this line item.

- **Payroll Taxes**: This practice is allocating 3.23% of total collections to Payroll Taxes. This is above the target of 2.5% by 0.73%, resulting in a score of +0.73 for this line item.

- **Fringe Benefits**: This practice is allocating 2.1% of total collections to Fringe Benefits. This is below the target of 2.5% by 0.4%, resulting in a score of −0.40 for this line item.

- **Total Payroll**: This category equals the total sum of all of the above line items. This practice is allocating 32.88% of total collections to Total Payroll. This is above the target of 30% by 2.88%, resulting in a score of +2.88 for this line item.

- **Lab Fees**: This practice is allocating 11.59% of total collections to Lab Fees. This is above the target of 9% by 2.59%, resulting in a score of +2.59 for this line item.

- **Dental Supplies**: This practice is allocating 6.79% of total collections to Dental Supplies. This is above the target of 5% by 1.79%, resulting in a score of +1.79 for this line item.

- **Doctor Salaries (owner plus associate dentists):** This practice is allocating 29.82% of total collections to Doctor Salaries. This is below the target of 30% by 0.18%. In the case of Doctor Salaries, no negative or positive points are given.
- **Advertising:** This practice is allocating 1.24% of total collections to Advertising. This is below the target of 4.5% by 3.26%, resulting in a score of −3.26 for this line item.
- **Other Minor Expenses:** This practice is allocating 0.31% of total collections to Other Minor Expenses. This is below the target of 2% by 1.69%, resulting in a score of −1.69 for this line item.
- **Other Expenses:** This practice is allocating 6.63% of total collections to Other Expenses. This is above the target of 5.5% by 1.13%, resulting in a score of +1.13 for this line item.
- **Insurance:** This practice is allocating 1.7% of total collections to Insurance. This is above the target of 1.5% by 0.2%, resulting in a score of +0.2 for this line item.
- **Legal and Accounting:** This practice is allocating .73% of total collections to Legal and Accounting. This is below the target of 1.5% by 0.77%, resulting in a score of −0.77 for this line item.
- **Office Expenses:** This practice is allocating 2.14% of total collections to Office Expenses. This is above

the target of 1.2% by 0.94%, resulting in a score of +0.94 for this line item.

- **Facility and Equipment:** This practice is allocating 5.61% of total collections to Facility and Equipment. This is below the target of 9% by 3.39%, resulting in a score of −3.39 for this line item.
- **Telephone:** This practice is allocating 0.76% of total collections to Telephone. This is below the target of 0.8% by 0.04%, resulting in a score of −0.04 for this line item.

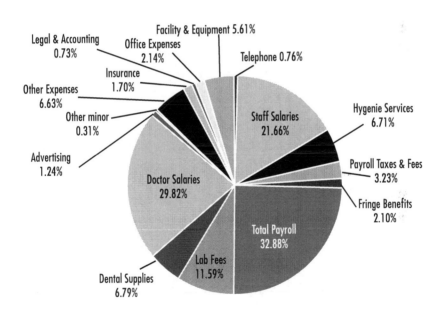

When all of the points from the above categories are added up, Dr. Jones' practice receives a score of 5.37. According to our classification, this practice "needs improvement."

The good news is—there are several areas of opportunity that, if focused upon, could help to get this practice's numbers in line. Even without addressing the issue of the overage in the total payroll, Dr. Jones can focus on controlling expenses in the areas of lab fees, dental supplies, "other expenses," insurance, and office expenses.

Getting these expenses down to the target percentages could potentially change this scorecard to −1.28 (Cruise Control) and drop the total office overhead from 69% to 62.35%, which would translate to an additional $9,468.73 of take-home profit for Dr. Jones.

With only expense reports from their CPA, profit and loss statements, and bank account records, Dr. Jones maybe aware that there are "holes in the bucket" but may not be able to locate exactly where those holes are. The solution to his frustration—the scorecard. Once he tracks his expenses via the scorecard, he can locate the holes and, more importantly, fix them. The big takeaway—the scorecard provides quick and easy clarity, demonstrating where changes need to be made in order to move any practice from loss to profitability.

CHAPTER 13:

CREATING A CULTURE OF EXCELLENCE

"Our number one priority is company culture. Our whole belief is that if you get the culture right, most of the other stuff like delivering great customer service or building a long-term enduring brand will just happen naturally on its own."
— Tony Hsieh CEO, Zappos.com

Every dental practice has a culture. The most basic definition of a practice culture is the collective personality, values, and attitudes of the owner and employees of the practice. The cultivation of a healthy practice culture can be one of the most important factors to the long-term success of a dental practice.

• • •

THE CULTURE OF EXCELLENCE FORMULA

As you can see in the following formula, I've defined a **"Culture of Excellence"** as a company's **Mission** plus its **Vision** plus its **Core Values.**

$$M+V+CV=CE$$

[**Mission + Vision + Core Values**] = **Culture of Excellence**

Whether or not you take the time to define, guide, and influence your practice's culture, one will develop. A culture that has not been intentionally designed and cultivated will simply reflect the personalities of each person on the team and his or her attitude toward his or her work and experience.

Your practice's culture will determine:

• The level of productivity and contentment of those on your team,

• The quality of care and customer service that your patients will experience while in your office, and

• The growth or stagnation of your business.

Because so much is riding on the culture of your practice, it makes sense to play an active role in its development.

Think about the possibility of creating a true **"Culture of Excellence"** within your organization. Each foundational component of your company's culture—Mission, Vision, and Core Values—serves an important and specific purpose that must be created with input from the entire team in order to be effective.

Much like the stool pictured here, your company's culture will be ineffective without a base of three strong legs.

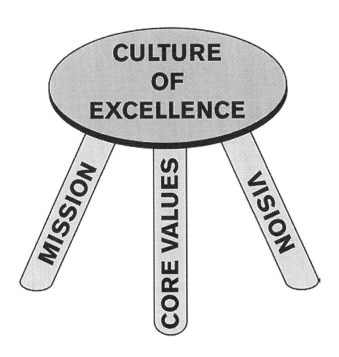

Culture of Excellence Three-Legged Stool

• • •

MISSION

A Mission Statement exemplifies the reason your company exists. One that is correctly written should be both persuasive and inspiring, while having the potential power to strategically drive your practice in the direction agreed upon by the team.

Here is a list of questions that will help you formulate an effective Mission Statement:

1. Why are you in business?

2. How would you like your patients to view you?

3. What level of service do you wish to provide?

4. Outside your core business, what else would you like your practice to be known for?

5. How are you different from your competitors?

Here are the three most important attributes of an effective Mission Statement:

1. Brief – The best Mission Statements are short and to the point.

2. Succinct – They should be very specific and not filled with overly used "buzzwords."

3. Actionable – They must be the framework of everything that is done at the practice.

. . .

MY COMPANY'S MISSION STATEMENT:

At Horizon Dental Group, our mission is to provide exceptional dental care to our patients while making a positive impact in our community.

As one of the main components of your company culture, your Mission Statement must be more than just words written on a piece of paper or that hang in your reception area. Your company's mission should serve as the framework that guides everything your business does and that allows each person on the team to remain clear and focused.

. . .

VISION

While the purpose of the Mission Statement is to clearly define why a company exists, a "Vision Statement" addresses where your company is going.

The vision statement serves as the inspiration for what you and the team strive to accomplish on a daily basis and guides your long-term strategic planning.

An effective Vision Statement must accomplish the following three things:

1. It must define what and where your practice aspires to be in the future.

2. It must be clear and visually descriptive.

3. It must be *big*, stretching the boundaries of possibility.

Writing a Vision Statement involves being able to visualize what the future is going to look like. Use the following questions as your guide:

1. What will the practice look like in five to ten years?

2. How will the community perceive us in five to ten years?

3. What will be our market position in five to ten years?

4. How will we remain true to our Mission Statement as we grow?

• • •

MY COMPANY'S VISION STATEMENT

At Horizon Dental Group, our vision is to deliver more exceptional dental care and community services than any other dental office in Central Arizona.

A strong Vision Statement should act as a beacon for your practice as you design and envision your ideal fu-

ture. It should work in concert with the Mission Statement and help to solidify a unified company culture.

• • •

CORE VALUES

A company's Core Values can be defined as the shared
ideas and principles that guide the behavior of every
person in your organization. Core Values should repre-
sent a combination of what your team finds most important in life. They help to clearly define your expectations for what is acceptable versus what is not allowed.
Core Values also declare and summarize how your company will treat its customers, vendors, community, and
internal team.

Here are several important questions to address:

- How committed are you to your Core Values?

- Does disregard for the agreed-upon Core Values
  result in dismissal?

- Are you willing to sacrifice monetary gain to
  protect your Core Values?

- Are you willing to hire based on culture fit first
  and industry qualifications second?

• • •

MY COMPANY'S CORE VALUES

1. Deliver exceptional patient care
2. Create an unforgettable patient experience
3. Build lifetime patient relationships
4. Cultivate respectful and honest communication
5. Practice kindness and understanding
6. Commit to continual growth and learning

As the third leg of our "Culture of Excellence" stool, our Core Values help to ensure that as we strive as an organization to live our Mission and Vision, we are not compromising the beliefs and standards of the team. If the Core Values of a company are not thoughtfully assembled with the input of the entire team, a Culture of Excellence can never be achieved. As your agreed-upon guiding principles, clearly defined Core Values create an atmosphere where decision making becomes much easier and straightforward.

• • •

YOUR IDEAL DENTAL PRACTICE

Once the foundational elements of Mission, Vision, Core Values, and Culture have been established, you can begin to engineer your ideal dental practice. In order to realize your dream business and work environment, you must have a crystal clear mental image of what it would look like. In order to be able to design and execute a definitive plan to create this practice, every last detail must be considered.

The "Perfect Day Exercise" will allow you to begin to visualize your ideal practice. It will help to identify areas within your practice that you might not have been consciously aware that you wanted to change. While answering the questions below, pretend there are absolutely no limitations regarding the facility, team, patients, procedures, and schedules. Remember that you want to try to visualize an absolutely "perfect day" that runs smoothly without any challenges or setbacks. Write the answers to the following questions on a separate piece of paper with as much detail as possible.

What time would you get up?

What would you do before you left for the office?

When you walk in the door of the office, what would it look like, smell like, and feel like?

How would you be greeted by your team?

How would the team be interacting with one another?

What time would you see your first patient?

What types of procedures would be on the schedule?

How would your team be dressed?

When you would overhear your staff answer the phone, what would it sound like?

How many patients would you see throughout the day?

How would you be greeted by your patients?

How would the day flow?

What would be your level of stress throughout the day?

What would your energy level be like throughout the day?

What types of comments would your patients be making to you throughout the day?

What type of feedback would you get from your team throughout the day?

What time would you leave the office at the end of the day?

How many hours would you work?

How would you feel physically at the end of the day?

How would you feel mentally and emotionally at the end of the day?

What would you do after you left the office?

(Extending out to Week, Month, and Year)

How many days would you be able to take off? Day/Week/Month/Year?

How much would you produce and collect? Day/Week/Month/Year?

How productive would your hygiene department be? Day/Week/Month/Year?

How many new patients would enter the practice?

Day/week/Month/Year?

Once you have answered all of the questions, compare your "perfect day" answers to your actual daily experience. This exercise will help to identify the areas with the biggest gap between your perfect day and your current reality. Taking the time to implement the systems covered in this book is the first step to systematically closing the gap between where you are and where you want to be.

CHAPTER 14:

THE ART OF DELEGATION

"No person will make a great business who wants to do it all himself or get all the credit."
— Andrew Carnegie

We all have the same twenty-four hours in a day. So why is it that some people get so much more done in the same period of time? The difference is that these high achievers have mastered the art of delegation.

Years ago, when I was juggling multiple practices, multiple associates, and multiple teams, I was working seventy to eighty hours per week and still didn't feel like I could keep up. At the time, I was doing everything from bookkeeping to general maintenance to employee management—on top of seeing a very full schedule of patients every day.

My days were chaotic and stressful. I initially believed that I was being a responsible business owner by saving money and doing everything that I could on my own. I also felt that I was the only person who could perform these tasks properly, and training another person to do them would be tedious and time-consuming.

I had put myself in a position where I was indispensable and irreplaceable. I felt as if the entire business would crumble in a day if I weren't there.

I was always the first one there and the last to leave. I insisted on making every decision myself and micromanaged every department in each office.

• • •

A LESSON IN TIME

During the same period of time, I had a meeting with one of my business coaches to look over the books. He commended me for the solid growth the company had experienced since the last time we met. When he asked how I was doing personally, I confided to him that I felt like a hamster on a wheel and that I could never seem to keep up—there just weren't enough hours in the day.

Without saying a word, he reached into his bricfcase and handed me a small stack of paper. At the top of each page was the title "Time Journal," followed by a blank space to fill in the day and date. Each hour of the day was printed vertically down the left-hand margin of the pages, and to the right was a space to make a short notation. He instructed me to write a brief summary of everything that I did from hour to hour for an entire week. He set up a follow-up appointment and told me to bring my completed "assignment" to the meeting.

When we reconvened a week later, he brought two highlighters with him, one yellow and the other blue. As we analyzed how I was spending each of my business days, he told me to highlight in yellow all of the tasks that I could pay someone else to do for less than one hundred dollars per hour. When I was finished, he asked me to highlight all of the remaining tasks in blue. As I flipped through the pages of my "Time Journal,"

I was shocked at how much yellow there was on each page. Then, he took out a blank piece of paper and drew a horizontal line across the top of the page and a vertical line down the middle, creating two columns. Above the left column he wrote *Low-Value Activities*. Above the right column, he wrote *High-Value Activities*. He instructed me to write out every task that appeared in the pages of my journal—yellow in the left column, blue on the right.

When I was done, we looked at the chart together.

He said, "Mark, by now, I'm sure you get the purpose of this exercise. I use highlighters because I want you to see the visual contrast between your high-value activities and your low-value activities. Right now, your low-value activities outnumber your high-value activities four to one. Filling your business days with low-value busy work is actually taking your time away from the activities that make you the most money. Find a way to get rid of the 'yellow' tasks from your day, and you'll work fewer hours and double your income."

He challenged me to start taking steps to delegate the activities from my left column and focus more on the items from my right column. He assured me that any cost associated with delegating these low-value activities would be recaptured by increased revenue that I would generate by focusing solely on my high-value activities. And more importantly, I'd be able to decrease my stress level and spend more time with my family. I'd finally get my life back.

I have to admit, I was skeptical at first. It didn't seem logical that I could actually pay someone else to do all of my busy work and make more money in the process. I was reluctant to relinquish control because I was convinced that nobody could do all of the tasks that I was doing to the level of my satisfaction.

I eased slowly into the transition of restructuring my days. I began by creating a written operational system for every aspect of each dental practice. Next, I defined the chain of command. Each department would have a supervisor, and each team member would have a defined set of tasks and expectations. The supervisor would hold each team member accountable for his or her tasks on a daily, weekly, and monthly basis. Updates from the supervisor to the office manager were made through a regularly scheduled in-person or virtual meeting. The office manager would then give me a short summary of each department on a weekly basis. The office manager was given the authority to make financial decisions up to a certain dollar amount and was instructed to contact me directly if there were a major issue. The protocol was presented to the team members, and they were asked to avoid bringing issues to me without first attempting a resolution with their supervisors. The new structure gave the supervisors a feeling of ownership over their departments and cultivated their leadership and problem-solving skills.

I immediately saved several hours per week that I had previously spent on management. I let my supervisors supervise and my managers manage, and my teams excelled in their areas of expertise.

Things actually started running more smoothly without my interference.

Streamlining the practice's operational systems and delegating tasks to my team was very effective for freeing up hours in my life, but I still felt as though I was wasting too much time doing low-level activities. I wanted to take my coach's advice and delegate all tasks that I could pay someone else to do for under one hundred dollars per hour.

I hired a personal assistant to help absorb many of the remaining tasks that were taking time away from a packed schedule. Her role was to help make my life less stressed and more organized by allowing me to focus only on my most high-value activities.

A partial list of her tasks included organizing and responding to e-mail; coordinating marketing campaigns; communicating with vendors; collecting and categorizing receipts for business expenses; making travel arrangements; shopping for business and personal items; picking up dry cleaning; making bank deposits; organizing and keeping track of continuing education credits; placing ads for open staff positions; coordinating marketing campaigns; and keeping personal and business schedules.

In the beginning, my assistant started part time, but as I started to learn how to effectively delegate, she quickly became a full-time employee. Since hiring her, my income has increased exponentially, and my quality of life has greatly improved.

Initially, when I made the commitment to begin delegating all of my low-value tasks to my team and to a personal assistant, my biggest reservation was the amount of time it would take to create the systems to be able to delegate efficiently. Looking back, I now realize that taking the time to set up the systems for delegation was the single biggest step in the growth and profitability of my business. I no longer feel frantic and disorganized, and I have the time and energy to do the things that are important to me. My creativity is no longer stifled, and I now have time to cultivate new projects and multiple streams of income.

· · ·

STEPS TO EFFECTIVE DELEGATION

1. Assign – Selecting the appropriate team member to complete your desired task is the first step in

the delegation process. These duties should be assigned according to each member's strengths.

2. Define the task or project – When you are delegating a task, it is important to deliver an exact definition of the task as well as the desired outcome. The project should be written to avoid any confusion or misunderstanding.

3. Verify – Once the team member has been assigned the task and it has been clearly defined, confirm that there is complete understanding.

4. Create a deadline- A task should never be assigned without a specific deadline. If it is a complex, multi-step project, several deadlines for tasks leading up to the completion of the project must be specified to ensure that the project is staying on schedule.

5. Design accountability – Having a clearly written task description with a deadline assigned to a qualified team member leaves little room for misunderstanding. Since the project is so well defined, accountability is very straightforward.

For many business owners, one of the hardest things to do is to delegate tasks that they know they can do by themselves. When the practice is young and the new dentist wants to learn how to perform certain tasks in order to better understand the business, doing low-value activities may be beneficial. But if these tasks are pulling the practice owner away from activities that are more valuable or more enjoyable, it's time to delegate.

CHAPTER 15:

THE POWER OF LEVERAGE

*"Give me a lever long enough and
I could move the world."*
- Archimedes

I have never regretted my choice to become a dentist. This profession has brought great people and amazing experiences into my life. But we all know that practicing dentistry is not without its challenges.

Maintaining the balance between effective practice management and exceptional clinical work can be stressful and exhausting—and generally speaking, as a profession, we are compensated well for it. But regardless of your income level, if you are a traditional dentist completely dependent upon a single income stream, you are simply "Trading hours for dollars." In other words, your income is directly proportionate to the number of hours that you spend working at the dental chair. Because there are only so many hours in the day, even the most efficient and highly productive dentists have an income ceiling.

When I was a young associate with two new cars, a mortgage, and a huge student loan, I struggled to make ends meet. I knew that I was going to have to increase my income somehow, so I did the one thing that I knew would get me there—I worked more hours. I put in ten-hour days and worked Saturdays to try to get a grasp on my personal overhead. The hard work eventually paid off, and I was slowly able to dig myself out of the hole.

Even back then, I knew that I wasn't going to be able to maintain the pace that I set for myself for very long without burning out. In an attempt to build multiple streams of passive income, I began building and acquiring multiple dental offices. What I quickly realized was that building and operating multiple dental offices created additional income, but it was far from passive!

Dealing with staff issues, operational management, and patient care created active, not passive, income. Simply put, I had built a business that required my constant presence and attention. I hadn't created life; I had created a job—a job that was very stressful and required a huge time commitment. Eventually, I finally did burn myself out and decided to sell four of the practices. After the offices farthest from my home were sold, I took the proceeds and went on a search for the elusive passive-income business.

In a word, I was dangerous. I had a large sum of money and was desperate to find a home for it, but I didn't have a strategy or a plan. I tried everything from real-estate investing to index option trading. I even bought a car wash. I was truly out of my element. I made a lot of expensive mistakes and ended up losing hundreds of thousands of dollars.

It was a very difficult time in my life. I had worked hard and sacrificed for years to build up a nice collection of successful dental practices that were generating millions of dollars. When I sold them, I expected to be able to roll the proceeds into a business that wouldn't require so much travel and personal time. But my haste and inexperience ended up costing me a big chunk of the proceeds from the practice sales.

THE ONE-INCH AD THAT CHANGED IT ALL

One of the few usable strategies that I picked up during my semester of "Practice Management" in dental school was to skim through the industry journals with a pair of scissors, cut out the useful articles, and discard the rest of the magazine. Then I'd place the clippings in categorized folders that I could reference and read when I had time. If I hadn't read the articles within two weeks, they hit the trash. This helped to combat my inner "pack rat" and kept me organized.

Although I almost never got all the way through the journals, on one particular day I made it all the way through a magazine to the classified ads section. While I was scanning through the collection of random ads, one headline caught my eye. It read: "*Start Your Own In-Office Dental Assisting School.*"

I had never heard of this concept before, but my mind immediately started racing. I had heard of the large national "institutes" and career training centers that taught certain vocations, but I had never heard of a dental-assisting school being held right inside a dental office. I thought the idea was ingenious. Who better to teach a dental assisting course than a dentist and the office personnel? We had the facility and expertise to pull this off.

• • •

GREAT CONCEPT—TERRIBLE PRODUCT

I immediately called the toll-free number listed in the classified ad and left a message requesting a call back and more information. I waited a day with no response. On my second attempt two days later, I left a message emphasizing that I was really interested and needed more information.

Finally, after another two days of waiting, I called again and finally got in touch with the owner of the company. He explained that yes, it was indeed possible to open a dental-assisting school inside a dental office. His company was offering detailed instructions for state licensure of an "accelerated post-secondary school." In addition, the company would provide all of the necessary teaching materials, including lectures, tests, quizzes, labs, and visual aids. Even though the company didn't offer any type of satisfaction guarantee, I decided to take the plunge. I gave him my credit card information and waited for the package to arrive.

When the box finally arrived two weeks later, I tore into it like a four-year-old on Christmas morning. I was shocked at what I found inside.

Basically, the entire program was two binders of scattered, disorganized information. The teaching materials included a series of outlines, visual aids, and tests. There were no lectures, and the labs were incomplete. If I were going to use any part of this curriculum, I was going to have to correct a lot of deficiencies.

The other binder contained a checklist and the phone number and website for the State Board of Post-Secondary Education. It would be up to my staff and me to research and assemble our application for licensure.

The curriculum that I had just spent thousands of dollars to purchase was completely unusable. Since I really believed in the concept, I decided that I wasn't going to give up. I threw the binders in the trash and resolved to create my own course. After all, I couldn't do any worse than the product that I had just pitched.

• • •

WRITE, RESEARCH, FILM, REPEAT

Even though I had recently simplified my life by selling four of my six dental practices, I was still working a full week between seeing patients and managing my two remaining offices.

After finally escaping the drudgery and stress of my eighty-hour weeks, I made a commitment to myself and my family that I would no longer be an absentee father or husband. Because of my personality, I knew that I had to be very careful not to get sucked back into my old habits by taking on a big project. After doing the preliminary research for what needed to be included in a dental-assisting-school curriculum, I realized that I had a long road ahead of me. I knew, however, that if I would be able to get to the other side of this challenge, I'd have a lifelong profitable side business that would generate income in my absence—a true passive-income machine.

In order to keep my family life unaffected by my new project, I structured my days the following way:

Monday – Thursday

5:30 a.m.: Wake up

5:45–6:30 a.m.: Workout in home gym

6:30–7:30 a.m.: Breakfast with Leslie and kids and get ready for work

7:30–8:00 a.m.: Commute to office

8:00 a.m.–4:45 p.m.: Dentistry

4:45 –5:15 p.m.: Commute home

5:15–8:00 p.m.: Family time (sporting activities, homework, etc.)

8:00 p.m.: Kids go to bed

8:00–9:00 p.m.: Time with Leslie

9:00 p.m.–1:00 a.m.: Write and research curriculum

In my previous life, I would have spent mornings, afternoons, and weekends laser-focused on a project like this until it was completed. I probably could have finished it in one-third the time if I had kept my eighty-hour-per-week schedule. But the whole idea behind the massive restructuring of my lifestyle was to get my life back. Yes, once the project was finished, I'd be able to reap the financial benefits and provide more for my family, but they needed me now. Even though I had to lose a bit of sleep, this new schedule kept my family and personal time sacred. I completed the entire dental-assisting-school curriculum after strictly adhering to this plan for one full year.

The finished curriculum, which includes six volumes, tests, and quizzes, detailed instructor and student lecture notes, a full complement of lab sessions, and videos of lectures and clinical procedures, was then presented to the Arizona State Board of Post-Secondary Education. The entire program, as well as our completed application, was approved on the first attempt—and the Horizon School of Dental Assisting was born.

One of the biggest deficiencies of the program that I had purchased one year earlier was a marketing element. Just like any other product or service, superior quality is irrelevant if nobody knows you exist. The marketing strategies that helped me build six successful dental practices in a short period of time are the same that I have used to consistently fill my dental-assisting-school sessions. While no single medium or advertisement is equally effective in every market, with testing, tracking, and multi-step marketing funnels, any school can become extremely profitable.

• • •

COAST TO COAST

Within a year of opening our first dental assisting school in my own dental office, I began offering our program to dentists throughout the United States. The program has been very well received by dentists from coast to coast, and as of this writing, our curriculum has been licensed to over one hundred different dental offices. When a doctor decides to join our network, he or she is assigned a personal liaison, who assists the new school owner through every stage of starting a new dental assisting school. The dentist or the dentist's assistant works hand in hand with the liaison through every step of the licensing and logistical setup of the new venture.

• • •

THE POWER OF LEVERAGE

Dentists are constantly inundated with new clinical techniques and gadgets designed to help them increase their revenue. If a dentist is simply trying to increase his or her income without considering the time that he or she spends at the chair, investing in new training and advanced equipment may make perfect sense. Using this tactic, however, a dentist will never break free from the hours for dollars scenario, and his or her income will always depend directly on the amount of time spent doing dentistry.

Most dentists don't realize that they already possess the assets that they need to create a significant secondary stream of income. In most cases, these valuable assets sit idle, never to realize their inherent value. Here is a short list of underutilized assets:

1. **Your facility** – As a business owner, you have intimate knowledge of the expense that it takes to construct and maintain a working dental office. Hundreds of thousands of dollars go into designing, building, and equipping your facility. This is obviously a justified expense because it is the location that is used to generate all of your revenue. But what happens after business hours? In most cases, once your dental operation shuts down, so does the facility. When you own an in-office dental-assisting school, you are able to leverage your facility to actually generate income in your absence. Everything that you need to train dental assistants is already available right in your facility. Nearly every other brick-and-mortar business must incur the expense of a facility build-out. Since you already have the perfect setup for this secondary business, there is no additional expense, which translates into lower operating expenses for

the owner and a greater percentage of profit.

2. **Your staff** – Have you ever hired a dental assistant with limited dental experience? In my offices, I hire for culture fit first and technical skills second. In other words, all of the dental experience in the world is insignificant if the new employee has a personality that does not mesh with the rest of the team. This has always been my philosophy, and it has served me well. So even before I started operating a dental assisting school out of my office, our entire team shared the responsibility of training the new team members. It is astonishing how quickly a complete neophyte can learn when mentored in the right environment. Your experienced team members are another underutilized asset that can be leveraged to generate additional revenue. Dental assistants or dental hygienists with at least two years of experience fit the ideal profile as dental-assisting school instructors. In most cases, they are enthusiastic about the opportunity to teach, pass on their craft, and earn extra money. This is a win–win–win scenario for all parties involved, because there is no need for the school owner to recruit outside help as instructors, the team members are happy to have the status as an educator as well as the extra income, and the students are getting an educational experience from experienced practitioners.

3. **Your degree** – The honest truth is that there is no one more qualified to own a dental assisting school

than a dentist. Your dental degree gives you all of the rights and privileges to practice dentistry, but it also gives you the necessary credentials to teach dental students, dental-hygiene students, and dental-assisting students at formal teaching institutions. I am personally passionate about teaching and have been a clinical instructor for many years. Unfortunately, selecting a career as a full-time educator did not offer the financial compensation that I was looking for. As a practicing dentist, you possess the necessary experience and credentials to open your own teaching facility. Students who obtain training from an in-office school will get a realistic perspective of how dentistry is practiced in the real world. You worked hard to get those three letters after your name. Are you fully leveraging them?

THE TRUTH ABOUT PASSIVE INCOME

When I went on my reckless search for a passive-income stream that would allow me to spend less time chair-side and more time living life and enjoying my family, I realized that there were very few opportunities that would deliver a safe and significant return. I looked into all types of franchises and investments. Most of what I found was very disappointing. Between build-out and franchise fees, fast-food restaurants required a huge up-front investment ($300K and up) and required a large time commitment. Additionally, it took up to ten years to break even on these types of businesses. Real estate and stock-market investment strategies tied up big chunks of money and took decades to realize a significant return.

For dentists, starting a dental-assistant school makes a lot of sense because it requires a minimal start-up investment, there is no need to pay for additional rent or build-out expense, and the break-even point usually takes place in less than one year. Due to the low overhead and relatively high ticket price (tuition can range from $2,500–$4,900 per student), a new school can potentially profit after its first session. Additionally, the entire operation can be run by the auxiliaries. This allows the doctor to experience increased income without spending any more time at the chair treating patients.

If you would like more information about starting your own in-office dental-assisting school, visit www.TeachDentalAssistants.com or call 1-888-275-9840.

CHAPTER 16:

A FEW WORDS FROM OUR CLIENTS

Mark,

Thank you for giving me the opportunity to share my experiences with you.

I have truly benefited from our friendship and your knowledge. You're a good man; you have admirable character with high moral values. The mentors you have surrounded yourself with are the elite of the elite. The core knowledge of dental practice management you have attained from these relationships is vast and impressive. Your ability and desire to pass on this knowledge and help others is a truly unique gift that I have eagerly accepted.

Your aid and guidance have helped me tremendously. My office is running more smoothly, and my stress level is greatly reduced. This has helped my overall mind-set. My staff and patients have noticed a change (for the better) in my attitude and behavior. One patient commented, "Dr. Flowers, I have never seen this side of you. I like it!" Noticeably, this has led to a better staff and a higher patient treatment plan acceptance rate. This in turn leads to more patient referrals and higher revenues, and the snowball grows....

Darren Flowers, DMD
Anthem, AZ

I met Dr Costes at an implant seminar. Right away, I knew that Mark was someone special, and that if I could ride on his coattails for a bit, my life would be different. My entire paradigm of dentistry has shifted with what I've learned from Mark. You really can have the best of both worlds by being a great clinician and a successful businessman!

I have started a dental assistant school and am having the most successful year of dentistry by leaps and bounds, while enjoying more time with my family and giving more back to the community.

Thanks, Mark, for all you've taught me through your Dental Success Summit and our Mastermind group! The paradigm shift has changed my life.

Jason W Lowry, DDS
Kingman, AZ

The Dental Success Summit is quite the eye-opener. It offers a detailed, tried, and tested plan to grow one's dental practice. Dr. Costes gives you all the keys to his own personal success. His referral generation, patient retention, marketing, and expense management strategies are brilliant. I definitely recommend the summit and personalized coaching from Dr. Costes to both successful and struggling practice owners alike!

Reddy Miranda
General Manager, Texas Dental

Dr. Mark Costes is an energetic go-getter who finds a problem and tackles it head-on. He talks about his childhood and goals, and one by one he has taken them by storm and conquered them. He is all about implementing systems and achieving success through helping people.

I have been a member of his Mastermind Group and Summit. What you first notice is how hard he works to make things go and his desire to help dentists become more independent. You leave with the feeling that he will knock you over with his energy. It's a great feeling. Hitch your wagon to his, and you will feel like he's given you a shot of Vitamin B-12.

Mark Caggiano, DDS
Seattle, WA

My wife, Sue, and I usually go to Arizona every February to see our son, Josh, his family, and our Wisconsin friends. I received a mailer on the Dental Success Summit, and the two-day lecture content looked intriguing to me, so we decided to go a day early. Wow! I was glad I took this opportunity to meet and learn from Dr. Mark Costes. Now this was a dental serendipity! Since I have been involved with several hands-on study clubs the last twenty-five years, I decided to join a Mastermind group to have support from Dr. Costes, Ashlee (his executive assistant), and other dentists in the group.

First, Dr. Costes upholds the standards and principles of our profession, knowing each dentist's quality of character is paramount to the success of his or her practices.

Secondly, his intensity is clearly visible as he teaches and mentors. He's driven by his goals and by achieving those goals. He knows that nothing great is ever accomplished without enthusiasm.

Thirdly, Dr. Costes's creativity is seen in the systems he has developed to benefit our practices. He sees the big picture as well as the details. I tend to procrastinate, and if you do as well, then be sure to make it to The Dental Success Summit, join a Mastermind group or get coaching from Dr. Costes. Your success will increase, resulting in greater fulfillment in dentistry.

Michael C Murat DDS, Fellow in the Academy of General Dentistry
The Dalles, OR

Dear Mark,

I just want to say thank you for helping my dad and me with our practice! After attending your Dental Success Summit in Scottsdale, we implemented many of the strategies and techniques you taught, and they have produced amazing results for us in a very short amount of time. We took home key points from all of your lectures and had a staff meeting that Monday. Our staff became very excited and involved in what we had to share with them. We definitely did not have a case of the "Next Seminar" syndrome, which usually happens after attending seminars. Our staff could see that we were more than ecstatic to adopt your advice and teachings into our practice, and they immediately were on board. We started an Internal Marketing Campaign modeled after the one you taught us, and the results have been incredible! Who knew that changing just a few things in the way we communicate with our patients would make such a huge difference? We cannot thank you enough.

In addition, your tips for Overhead Control and Systems Implementation were just what we needed in the management aspect of our practice. As we are rapidly expanding, our overhead started to increase in the same way. With your "Cash Flow Tracker" tool, we are now able to keep our expenses in check while still growing at an astounding pace. You made implementing systems in our office something that we could actually introduce, execute, and maintain. Whereas before, we could introduce systems, but the execution and mostly the maintaining aspects were eventually lost.

You know how to connect with the dentist and understand the business/management aspect of dentistry better than most in our field. In addition, you can relay information that is sometimes difficult to comprehend or grasp in such a simple and straightforward way. It makes actually using all of the information we learn in seminars a reality.

We cannot thank you enough for all of the help you have given us through attending your Dental Success Summit. You have made such an incredibly positive impact not only on our practice but with us and the people we associate with. We would *highly recommend any dental professional and his or her staff to attend at least one of your Dental Success Summits and coaching programs. The information and knowledge you will gain is invaluable. We cannot wait to continue to work with you and your amazing team in reaching goals in our practice that we never thought we would be able to achieve. You guys are the best!*

Som Gupta, DDS & Sumit Gupta, DDS Pittsburgh, PA

I first met Mark Costes a couple of months before his Success Summit. He was with a group of dentists at an implant seminar and was trying, like the rest of us, to improve his skills in placing implants and in the systems associated with making that a routine procedure.

After talking with him a bit, I realized that this guy was a chairside dentist who had figured out how to build dental practices. He had built six and had a reliable system for doing this.

After attending the Success Summit, I was even more convinced that I wanted to try his system. He had writtenit all down in what is almost a cookbook system—the "Dental Practice Accelerator." Best of all, it included a lot of things that I was already doing but had never systematized in order so that I could see maximum benefit from them—things like giving a really great new-patient experience, thanking referrals with a note and a gift, sending cards to acknowledge big events in patients' lives, donating both time and money to worthwhile community organizations, and reactivating patients who hadn't been back to our office for a while. But because of the way the systems are set up, each of these activities builds on the others, and the whole is greater than the sum of the parts. It all seemed so simple and made such sense. I've been in practice twenty-five years—why didn't I think of this?

As I was sitting in the seminar, knowing that I wanted to do this, my next thought was, "How am I going to implement this and hold myself accountable?" I've been to plenty of seminars and have only used a fraction of the information presented because I just lost steam in trying to get things implemented. Enter—the Elite Practice Mastermind Group. Mark was putting together a group of dentists to work together on this and other things to help grow their practices. I signed up and went back to Arizona the next month to attend the first meeting. It was great! There were ten participants and everyone had a really great attitude about helping each other work through practice issues so that all of us could get past our blockages and grow. Not everyone practiced in the same area of the country, had the same type of practice, or even wanted the same type of practice growth. But together, we seemed to have the answers to each other's practice problems.

I guess that's the beauty of a mastermind group.

My experience with Mark, his organization, the Success Summit, and the Elite Practice Mastermind Group has been very positive. It is one of the best things I've done for my practice/business. It has been just the right situation at just the right time. I'd recommend any of his books, systems, or seminars without hesitation. He's taken the guesswork out of *practice growth and has made it into a turnkey system—just implement and go!*

Aaron Nicholas, DDS
Burtonsville, MD

FREE 30 MINUTE STRATEGY SESSION WITH DR. MARK COSTES

If you are ready to take your practice to the next level, let's schedule a time to talk. During the call, we can discuss the biggest challenges and opportunities within your practice and strategize a plan to increase your profitability while decreasing your stress and the amount of time spent at the office.

I want you to regain your passion for dentistry!

To take advantage of this offer, simply email our headquarters at: info@PillarsOfDentalSuccess.com or call (800) 585-5706.

If you'd like to receive our free practice building articles and videos, log on to

www.PillarsOfDentalSuccess.com

All the Best,

Mark Costes. DDS

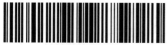

Made in the USA
San Bernardino, CA
24 February 2016